Ultrasound in Emergency Care

Ultrasound in Emergency Care

Edited by

Adam Brooks

*Division of Traumatology and Surgical Critical Care,
University of Pennsylvania, USA*

and

Jim Connolly

Newcastle General Hospital, Newcastle-upon-Tyne, UK

and

Otto Chan

Royal London Hospital, London, UK

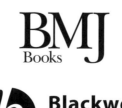

BMJ Books

Blackwell Publishing

First published 2004

Library of Congress Cataloguing-in-Publication Data

Ultrasound in emergency care / edited by Adam Brooks and Jim Connolly, and Otto Chan.
     p. ; cm.
ISBN 0-7279-1731-5 (alk. paper)
     1.   Medical emergencies—Ultrasonic imaging, 2.   Emergency medicine—Diagnosis.
[DNLM: 1.   Wounds and Injuries—ultrasonography. 2.   Emergency Treatment—methods. WO 700
U47 2004] I.   Brooks, Adam, 1969- II.   Connolly, Jim, 1964– III.   Chan, Otto
     RC86.7.U45 2004
     616.07′543—dc22   2004009786

A catalogue record for this title is available from the British Library

Set by SIVA Math Setters, Chennai, India
Printed and bound in Spain by GraphyCems, Navarra

Commissioning Editor: Mary Banks
Development Editor: Nic Ulyatt
Production Controller: Kate Charman

For further information on Blackwell Publishing, visit our website:
http://www.blackwellpublishing.com

The publisher's policy is to use permanent paper from mills that operate a sustainable forestry policy, and which has been manufactured from pulp processed using acid-free and elementary chlorine-free practices. Furthermore, the publisher ensures that the text paper and cover board used have met acceptable environmental accreditation standards.

Contents

Contributors

Dominic Barron
Department of Radiology, Leeds Teaching Hospital NHS Trust, Leeds, UK

Christopher Boyd
Department of Radiology, Leeds Teaching Hospital NHS Trust, Leeds, UK

Adam Brooks
Division of Traumatology and Surgical Critical Care, University of Pennsylvania, USA

Otto Chan
Department of Radiology, Royal London Hospital, London, UK

Jim Connolly
Emergency Medicine, Newcastle General Hospital, Newcastle-upon-Tyne, UK

Robert Cooper
Department of Radiology, Northern General Hospital, Sheffield, UK

Ben Davies
Cardiothoracic Surgery, Northern General Hospital, Sheffield, UK

Anthony J Dean
Department of Emergency Medicine, University of Pennsylvania Medical Center, USA

Scott A Dulchavsky
Wayne State University School of Medicine, Detroit, Michigan and National Aeronautics and Space Administration, Johnson Space Center, Houston, Texas, USA

Simon England
Department of Radiology, Sunderland Royal Infirmary, Sunderland, UK

Douglas R Hamilton
Wyle Laboratories, Houston, Texas, USA

Susie Hewitt
Emergency Medicine, Derby Royal Infirmary, Derby, UK

Leonard J King
Department of Radiology, Royal Hospital Haslar, Gosport, Hampshire, UK

Andrew Loughney
Department of Obstetrics and Gynaecology, Royal Victoria Infirmary, Newcastle-upon-Tyne, UK

Michael R Marohn
Department of Surgery, Uniformed Services University of the Health Sciences, Bethesda, Maryland, USA

Richard G McWilliams
Department of Radiology, Royal Liverpool Hospital, Liverpool, UK

Ali Naraghi
Department of Radiology, Royal London Hospital, London, UK

M Gage Oschner
Division of Trauma and Critical Care, Memorial Medical Center, Savannah, Georgia, USA

Ashot Sargysan
Wyle Laboratories, Houston, Texas, USA

Stephen Stirgess
Department of Obstetrics and Gynaecology, Royal Victoria Infirmary, Newcastle-upon-Tyne, UK

Daniel K Vining
Department of Emergency Medicine, University of Pennsylvania Medical Center, USA

David Wherry
Department of Surgery, Uniformed Services University of the Health Sciences, Bethesda, Maryland, USA

James L Williams
Orthopaedic Trauma Fellow, Auckland City Hospital, Auckland, New Zealand

Preface

Ultrasound is a well accepted modality in everyday clinical practice. However, it is only during the last decade that it has been introduced into the emergency room in order to answer highly specific questions in the management of critically ill patients. Focussed ultrasound has rapidly developed from the original evaluation of abdominal trauma by surgeons and emergency physicians, to include a range of focussed applications in both the injured and acutely ill patient.

The contributors to this book are at the forefront of innovation and teaching in this field. Their work has allowed us to produce a book that covers a wide range of indications for focussed ultrasound where each application aims to answer highly specific questions for the management of the patient. We hope that this book will help those involved in the emergency care of patients to develop a portfolio of focussed ultrasound techniques relevant to their day to day practice.

Like any new skill, we owe it to our patients to ensure we are adequately trained and a discussion chapter at the end of this publication reviews the current American system and gives a vision of future accreditation and training in this field for UK readers.

We are grateful to all the contributors for their drive, vision, and enthusiasm in developing focussed emergency ultrasound, which will undoubtedly benefit the most ill and injured patients. We are particularly indebted to Professor David Wherry for his vision and encouragement.

Adam Brooks
Jim Connolly
Otto Chan

Ultrasound in Emergency Care CD Rom

Features

- Video clips and additional ultrasound images
- Ultrasound in Emergency Care PDF eBook
- Bookmarked and hyperlinked for instant access to all headings and topics
- Fully indexed and searchable text – just click the "Search Text" button

Instructions for use

The CD Rom should start automatically upon insertion, on all Windows systems. The menu screen will appear and you can then navigate by clicking on the headings. If the CD Rom does not start automatically upon insertion, please browse using "Windows Explorer" and double-click the file "BMJ_Books.exe".

Tips

The viewable area of the PDF ebook can be expanded to fill the full screen width by hiding the bookmarks. To do this, click and hold on the divider in between the bookmark window and the main window, then drag it to the left as required.

By clicking once on a page in the PDF eBook window, you "activate" the window. You can now scroll through pages using the scroll-wheel on your mouse, or by using the cursor keys on your keyboard.

Note: the Ultrasound in Emergency Care PDF eBook is for search and reference only and cannot be printed.

Troubleshooting

If any problems are experienced with use of the CD Rom, please send an email to the following address stating the problem you have encountered: cdsupport@bmjbooks.com

1 History of ultrasound in emergencies

BEN DAVIES, ADAM BROOKS

Objectives
- To review the background to the development of ultrasound
- To review the introduction of diagnostic ultrasound into emergency care

Introduction

Since the discovery of the piezo-electric effect in the late 19th century, ultrasound (US) has evolved from a tool for military maritime echo-location into a diagnostic medical modality in its own right. US has expanded across many disciplines including vascular surgery, obstetrics and gynaecology, urology, cardiology, breast, musculoskeletal, and emergency medicine, and is widely employed both in image acquisition and interventional roles.

Origins of ultrasound

Early acoustic work by philosophers and scientists such as Pythagoras, Aristotle, and Galileo laid down the fundamental principles concerning the physical properties and characteristics of sound. It is from these beginnings that medical ultrasound took its origins. In the 19th century physicists moved on to more sophisticated experiments to calculate the speed of sound underwater and subsequently attempt to map the ocean floor. In 1822 Daniel Colladen estimated the speed of sound using an underwater bell in Lake Geneva, producing a figure (1435 m/s) not dissimilar to its accepted value today.

The discovery of the piezo-electric effect by the Curie brothers in 1880 proved pivotal in facilitating greater understanding and development in the field. In short, they recognised that an electrical potential could be produced when mechanical pressure was exerted on a quartz crystal and that likewise, applying an electrical charge was found to make the crystal vibrate and produce sound waves. They concluded that if these could be accurately harnessed with an appropriately constructed timing device and display, then the behaviour of sound waves in various media could be visually demonstrated.

Two significant events, the sinking of the Titanic in 1912 and the advent of the first world war, provided further impetus for the development of maritime echo-location in both surface ships and underwater navigation by the first submarines. In 1915, Langévin, working in Paris, began experimenting with high-frequency acoustic waves and quartz resonators. This work culminated in the development of an echosounding device, which he termed a "hydrophone", that could detect underwater obstacles be they natural hazards or submarines. Indeed, by the 1930s, many French ocean-going liners were fitted with so-called SONAR (sound navigation and ranging).

Meanwhile in the United Kingdom, United States of America and the Soviet Union ultrasonic detectors were employed on dry land to assess the integrity of various metal constructions including ships' hulls and battle tanks, a technique pioneered by Sokolov in 1928.

The second world war saw significant advances in sonar, radar (radio direction and ranging) and electronics, with the first digital computer built at Bletchley in 1944. This was followed by the invention of the transistor in 1947, which allowed miniaturisation of electronic devices that had hitherto relied on bulky valves.

Initially used for therapeutic means in the medical setting, the heating and disruptive effects of ultrasound were used on living tissue for physiotherapy and rehabilitation. William Fry and Russell Meyers, neurosurgeons from the Universities of Illinois and Iowa respectively, used ultrasonic probes in the 1940s to destroy the basal ganglia of Parkinson's sufferers in an attempt to palliate some of the more distressing symptoms.

At the same time, the Dussik brothers in Austria were attempting to localise brain tumours and the ventricles by transmitting ultrasound beams through the head using transducers strapped to either side of the skull. In hindsight, many of the images they obtained may have been artefactual but it nevertheless opened people's eyes to the potential of ultrasound as a diagnostic modality.

Another pioneer, Ludwig, a physician from Pennsylvania working at the Michigan Institute of Technology, demonstrated gallstones for the first time and his team went on to develop two-dimensional ultrasound image formation.

The immediate post-war period saw new advances in materials and electronics. Newer piezoceramics provided better sensitivity, frequency handling, efficiency, and sizing considerations and ushered in the modern era of ultrasonics, fuelling applications in medicine, science, and industry.

Japanese researchers began to further explore diagnostic medical applications, building the first model with A-mode presentation – blips on an oscilloscope screen – which was followed by work on B-mode presentation of two-dimensional, gray-scale imaging.

The first practical human B-mode scanner was manufactured in 1957 by Tom Brown and Ian Donald in Scotland, and used for abdominal and obstetric imaging. Donald and his group had started out using metal-flaw detectors to investigate abdominal and pelvic masses and despite many doubters their work evolved into the two-dimensional grey-scale representation we recognise today.

From these beginnings grew the sophisticated diagnostic modality that is used today for diagnostic and interventional procedures. Technological and software developments have permitted improvements in image quality, miniaturisation, and true portability, facilitating ultrasound's application at the bedside and in previously impossible situations including remote field and mass casualty work.

Emergency ultrasound

The introduction of ultrasound into the acute management of patients has occurred in a non-coordinated fashion. Although radiologists have been using US for many years it is the dissemination of the technology into the hands of different specialties that has brought about the

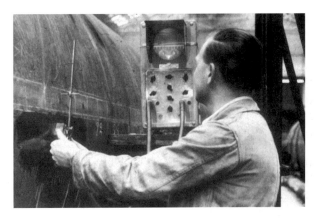

Figure 1.1 A Henry Hughes Mk 2 flaw detector like this was used by Donald in his first experiments.

expansion of the use of US in emergency care. Emergency ultrasound for the acute assessment of patients, performed by non-radiologists, has been established longest in obstetrics and gynaecology where it is valuable in the evaluation of ectopic pregnancy, assessment of the fetal heartbeat and fetal viability amongst other applications. Numerous other specialties use ultrasound to augment clinical decision making in both the acute and elective setting, for example echocardiography, assessment of aneurysms, intra-operative ultrasound, etc.

The ultrasound examination performed for acute care by emergency physicians or other non-radiologists is distinctly different from those performed in the radiology department. It is usually performed at the bedside simultaneously with clinical examination, resuscitation, or procedure. It has been described as an extension of the palpating hand and a "visual" stethoscope during the physical examination, providing further anatomic and functional information to supplement other clinical findings. In performing such examinations, the physician does not nor should not seek to replace the more detailed, formal examination performed by radiologists but usually attempts to answer a single, focused, pertinent clinical question within minutes. For example a group of trained non-radiologists have been shown to be as good as radiologists in a focused investigation to detect gallstones in patients with right upper quadrant pain. The history of non-radiologist performed emergency ultrasound is most clearly charted by the development of ultrasound for trauma.

Trauma ultrasound

The use of ultrasound for traumatic torso injury began in Europe and spread to North America in the 1990s where it was taken up enthusiastically, to the extent that it has virtually eliminated the initial use of diagnostic peritoneal lavage (DPL) at many trauma centres in the United States.

Initial cadaveric studies by Goldman and others in 1970 demonstrated the ability of ultrasound to detect as little as 100 ml of free fluid in dependent areas of the abdomen and proposed its use for the diagnosis of ascites. Following this, Kristensen in Germany published the first case report documenting the use of ultrasound in the assessment of a trauma patient. Subsequent German studies described its routine use in the emergent setting. Meanwhile in the USA, Asher's prospective study from 1976 demonstrated a sensitivity of 80% in 70 patients with suspected splenic injury.

Chambers and Pilbrow suggested US as a non-invasive alternative to DPL and highlighted the importance of the abdomen's dependent areas in the diagnosis of haemoperitoneum. With the trauma patient lying supine, free fluid gravitates naturally to the same dependent areas, namely adjacent to the diaphragm and in the pelvic sump. Liu and co-workers demonstrated equivalence between US, DPL and CT in a prospective study, suggesting that all were complementary but also sounding a cautionary note about the potential for US to miss bowel injuries when used in isolation.

Grace Rozycki, a trauma surgeon based in Atlanta, Georgia, USA, was the lead of a prospective landmark study where patients had US examination followed by DPL, CT or surgical exploration. Ultrasound was shown to have a 79% sensitivity and 96% specificity. This study focused the US investigation on the detection of free fluid as opposed to solid organ injury *per se* and was the first to show that non-radiologists (trauma surgeons or surgical residents) could reliably detect haemoperitoneum using a focused US protocol in any of the pericardial sac and three dependent abdominal areas: right-upper quadrant, left-upper quadrant and pouch of Douglas. Her group coined the term FAST (focussed assessment with sonography for trauma) and developed the concept of the modality acting as an adjunct to clinical examination.

Trauma ultrasound has continued to evolve and become accepted as an appropriate investigation for the trauma patient. Focused techniques have also been developed to expand FAST to assess for haemothorax and pneumothorax as well as cardiac tamponade in penetrating trauma.

Summary

Ultrasound plays an increasing role in the assessment of the acute patient and is now widely accepted in emergency medicine. The American College of Emergency Physicians (ACEP) has stated, "Emergency physicians regardless of practice, location or type, should be encouraged to adopt this extraordinarily useful modality in the leading decade of the 21st century." With the current level of technological development, it is a modality superbly amenable to use at the point of care and its application in emergent situations by non-radiologists with appropriate training is likely to increase.

2 The physics of ultrasound

JIM CONNOLLY

Objectives
- To understand the basics of ultrasound physics
- To understand how this is used to create images
- To define and understand common terminology
- To understand the physics behind the Doppler principle
- To understand safety issues

Introduction

Over recent years there has been an explosion in applications for which ultrasound can be used across an increasing number of specialties. In order to obtain the best image possible, a basic understanding of ultrasound physics is vital to understand how images are produced and to enable manipulation of these images. The following chapter is designed to give the reader a basic understanding of ultrasound physics, so that they can get started in scanning. The reader is encouraged to refer to other more exhaustive texts (see further reading.)

The physics of sound

Ultrasound is, as the name suggests, very high-pitched sound (defined as > 20 000 Hz), which is above the limits of human hearing. Sound travels in longitudinal waves by alternately compressing and relaxing (rarefaction) the tissues it travels through. Because of this it needs a medium to travel through (sound will not travel in a vacuum). The frequency of the sound is how many of these waves (cycles) appear per second. The waves, as previously stated, are made up of alternating compressions and rarefactions of the medium that the sound is travelling through (Figure 2.1), caused by molecular vibrations in the medium. A single cycle encompasses one compression and one rarefaction. The period is the time it takes for one cycle to pass a point (for example a 10 MHz frequency would take 0·1 microseconds to pass).The maximal deflection from the resting state of the wave is referred to as the amplitude.

$$\text{Wavelength} = \frac{1}{\text{Frequency}}$$

Amplitude is different from the intensity. The intensity is the amount of energy passing through a given area (mwatt/cm^2), and so as the area through which a set amount of sound passes is decreased so the power (intensity) rises (focusing).

Ultrasound physics

The sound waves used in ultrasound are between 2 and 10 MHz (2 to 10 000 000 cycles per second). Understanding what can happen to these waves is simple if they are thought of as sound waves. Sound waves travel at different velocities through different media (Table 2.1).

When sound strikes an interface between two different media it can be *reflected, refracted or scattered* (Figure 2.2). By detecting the returning sound waves an image can be created. The amount of reflection is shown by the brightness of dots on the screen, black for no echo (*anechoic*), white for a strong echo (*hyperechoic*), whilst the time taken for the sound to return can be used to represent its distance from the surface.

Table 2.1 shows the speed of sound in various tissues (*acoustic velocity*), which is relatively independent of the frequency of the sound wave. As can be seen in the majority of soft tissues this varies little and so these tissues appear as differing shades of grey.

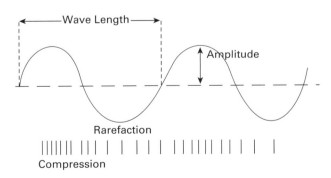

Figure 2.1 Wavelength/compressions, rarefactions, and amplitude.

Table 2.1   Speed of sound in common biological media

Material	Speed (metres per second)
Air	330
Water	1480
Bone	4080
Liver	1550
Kidney	1560

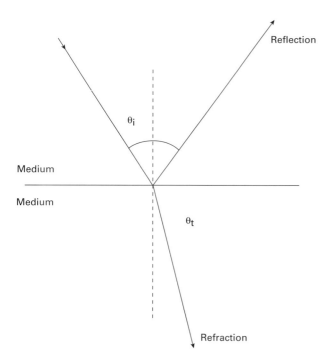

Figure 2.2   Reflection and refraction.

Reflection, refraction and scatter

Reflection is when the waves are returned from the interface between two surfaces. The angle of reflection is equal to the angle of incidence. At most boundaries very little of the sound is reflected back.

Refraction occurs when the wave passes obliquely through two differing media, and is caused by the fact that sound has different impedances in media. It is governed by Snell's law.

$$\sin\theta_t = (c2/c1) \times \sin\theta_i$$

θ_t = transmit angle
θ_i = incident angle
c = speed of travel of sound in media

Ultrasound reflects at boundaries between tissues, and the amount of reflection is dependent upon the differences between the media.

Reflections from a large smooth surface (for example diaphragm) are called *specular reflections*. However if the surface is rough or the size of the surface is of similar or a smaller size to the wavelength the sound will be *scattered*. This is of use in scanning as it allows the tissue between boundaries to be visualised.

Sound waves that are transmitted will then come to other interfaces and the process will be repeated so that different interfaces will be reflected back at differing depths. The machine is able to calculate these distances based upon the speed of sound and the time taken for the reflection to return and so represent them as different depths on the screen.

Tissues differ greatly in their ability to transmit sound waves. Bone is a poor transmitter and thus reflects strong signals back. Because of this it casts an *acoustic shadow* that makes it difficult to see anything behind it. Air is also a poor conductor (this is why a coupling gel is needed on the skin – to eliminate air).

Other tissues like soft tissue (liver, spleen, etc.) transmit sound well (*hypoechoic*). Fluid (blood, ascites, etc) is considered *anechoic* as it transmits very well and because of this property objects viewed behind a fluid filled space receive increased sound and so appear brighter (*acoustic enhancement*). Air filled tissues (for example lung, bowel) transmit poorly (*hyperechoic*) producing multiple echoes.

The effect of changing frequency

High frequencies produce much better *resolution* (the ability to detect two separate objects) but do not penetrate well, whereas the reverse is true of lower frequencies. Thus different frequency probes (or an electronic switching system within the machine) are required to image different structures (Table 2.2).

The higher the frequency the less it can penetrate. The development of higher frequency probes has allowed the development of soft tissue radiology, as it has permitted high resolution imaging of relatively superficial structures.

Table 2.2 Frequency of probes needed for different structures

Frequency	Application
7·5MHz	Breast, neck subcutaneous tissues
5·0MHz	Small adult, paediatric abdomen
3·5MHz	Adult abdomen and chest
2·5MHz	Large adult abdomen and chest

Important definitions

Impedance

This is the resistance of tissues to compression and rarefaction and is equal to the

Density × speed in tissue

It is the difference in impedance between tissues that defines what happens to the sound, that is if it is reflected or refracted.

Attenuation

This is the decrease in strength of a signal (amplitude) as it passes through a medium and is caused by a mixture of absorption, scatter, reflection, and divergence of the sound beam. As the frequency increases so does attenuation, almost linearly, which is why higher frequency waves penetrate poorly.

Because of this characteristic the machinery is designed to have ways of compensating, either by time gain compensation or depth gain compensation, so that deeper structures can be visualised (see Chapter 3).

Frequency and resolution

Higher frequencies give better resolution (but penetrate less). For example a 3 MHz probe has an axial resolution of 1·1 mm but a 10 MHz probe can resolve up to 0·3 mm. The returning mechanical waves are converted back into electrical signals that are displayed on a screen; the size (amplitude) of the returning echo dictates the brightness of the dots:

*   strong reflections = WHITE, for example diaphragm, bone, gallstones
*   weaker = GREY, for example most solid organs, thick fluid

*   no reflection = BLACK, for example fluid, urine, blood.

The position for each of the dots is also shown on the screen, and represents its depth and position relative to the probe.

Axial resolution – this is how close two objects can be along the axis of a beam and still be detectable. It is affected by the frequency.

Lateral resolution – the ability to resolve two objects parallel to the beam. It is affected by the bandwidth.

Contrast resolution – the ability to resolve two adjacent objects of similar intensity and reflectivity as different objects.

Temporal resolution – the ability to locate the position of a moving structure at particular instants in time, and is dependent on the frame rate.

Absorption

As sound passes through various media it is absorbed and energy is lost, mostly as heat. This is directly proportional to the frequency of the sound.

The production of ultrasound waves

These high-speed sound waves are produced by changing electrical energy into mechanical energy using piezo-electric crystals. These crystals are able to change shape as a current is applied across them. They can also change mechanical energy back to electrical energy so that images can be created. Millions of pulses are sent and received each second (*pulse echo method*) and during any one second the probe is only transmitting for less than 1% of the time (*the duty factor*); the rest of the time it is acting as a receiver. This is important, as otherwise echo detection would not be possible.

A *pulse* is made up of a number of cycles (typically two or three in normal ultrasound and up to 10 in Doppler measurements). The *pulse repetition frequency* is the time from the beginning of one pulse to the beginning of another. It is by altering the thickness of the crystal that the frequency can be altered.

Each probe contains many of these crystals (*array*) and they fire off at slightly different times (*phased array*).

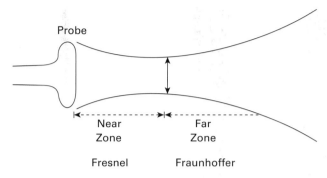

Figure 2.3 Beam characteristics.

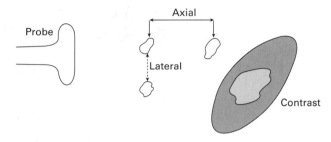

Figure 2.4 Different types of resolution.

Beam properties

The transducer can produce a number of different types of beam depending on how the piezo-electric crystals are arranged in the transducer and the wavelength of the sound:

- *linear array* – creates a rectangular image
- *sector array* – creates a fan type view. This is useful for echocardiography for imaging between the ribs
- *annular array* – creates a circular image best exemplified by trans-vaginal and trans-rectal probes.

The beam produced has three distinct areas.

- *Near* – an area where the beam diameter decreases as it moves away from the probe. This is also known as the *Fresnel zone*.
- *Focal zone* – the area where the beam diameter is at its most narrow. This is the area where it is most focused.
- *Far zone* – as the beam gets further and further away the beam width starts to increase. This is also known as the *Fraunhoffer zone*. It is obviously more difficult to differentiate two objects (resolution) in this zone.

Components of an ultrasound system

Transducer

As described previously this is the part of the probe that houses the crystals that transduce (or changes) energy between electrical and mechanical.

Pulse generator

This produces and delivers voltage to the transducer, which is then changed into mechanical energy.

Gain controls

These allow tuning of the signals to improve different areas of the image. For example, far gain will enhance distant echoes and so improve the imaging of deeper structures. Time gain compensation will increase the amplitude of signals with time from pulse transmission and so also improve images in the deeper structures.

Central processing unit (CPU)

This is the brain of the system. It is this area of the machine that acts as a computer and performs all the calculations needed to produce an image.

Transducer pulse controls

These can change the amplitude, frequency and duration of pulses.

Display

This is the screen where the images are displayed.

These will be described in more detail in the next chapter.

Image Display

The images can be displayed in different ways: *A-mode, B-mode real time* or *M-mode*.

A-mode (amplitude mode)

A-mode shows images as peaks or blips on an oscilloscope corresponding to the amplitude of the returning signal. The distance between these can be measured.

B-mode (brightness mode)

The signals returning are represented by individual points on the screen. The brightness of each dot represents the strength (amplitude) of the returning signal. This is used to create a two-dimensional image (*tomogram*) that shows all the tissues the sound waves pass through (like taking a single slice through a structure). It can easily be imagined that if this was repeated in rapid succession then a *real time* picture could be created.

M-mode (motion mode)

This is when pulses of ultrasound are used to detect and record motion. Motion is displayed as a function of depth against time, motion towards being positive and away negative. It is best exemplified by the images obtained during echocardiography.

Doppler

The Doppler effect, first described by the Austrian physicist Christian Johann Doppler (1805–53) in 1842, describes the effect of motion on the reflected frequency of waves, and originally described the light waves emitted from stars. An object moving towards a point will reflect back signals at a higher frequency and vice versa.

The classic description is that of an ambulance siren moving towards and then away from somebody standing still. As the siren comes closer the pitch is raised but goes lower as the vehicle moves away. The amount of change in the frequency (*Doppler shift*) is proportional to the speed of the object and so a measurement of flow can be made.

$$Df = \frac{2fV \cos q}{c}$$

V = velocity
Df = Doppler shift
c = speed of sound
q = angle between beam and blood

The major reflectors are the blood cells. The electronics allow the detection of the difference between normal reflections and reflections that have undergone Doppler shift.

As the cosine of 90 degrees is zero it can be appreciated that a Doppler probe placed vertically to the flow will show no Doppler shift (and hence no flow). In general the probe should be held at < 60 degrees to the flow as the cosine curve has a steeper curve greater than this.

There are several different ways in which the Doppler image can be depicted.

- *Colour Doppler* gives an estimate of flow rate and represents it as a colour against a grey background (red towards, blue away). It is important to appreciate that *the colour display represents direction of flow and not arterial and venous blood.*
- *Pulsed Doppler* allows a sample to be taken by a quick pulse of sound, allowing a graphic representation of flow.
- *Power Doppler* shows the power of the Doppler signal as opposed to the amount of Doppler shift.

Risks of ultrasound

Epidemiological studies have yet to show any human risk in the operating range of modern ultrasound machines, but it remains prudent to keep an open mind when using ultrasound.

In general ultrasound can produce the effects of cavitation and heating.

The American Institute of Ultrasound in Medicine (AIUM) noted

> no confirmed biological effects on patients or instrument operators caused by exposure at intensities typical of present diagnostic ultrasound, although the possibility exists that such biological effects may be identified in the future. Current data indicates that benefits to the patient of prudent use of diagnostic ultrasound outweighs the risks, if any, that may be present.[1]

In general the sonographer should adhere to the ALARA principle (As Low As Reasonably Achievable) by using the machine for as short a time as necessary to achieve an image, by minimising the machine output when obtaining the view, and using only when medically indicated.

Crucial to this is keeping the intensity (the amount of power passing through a given area) as low as possible. The *temporal peak intensity* is the highest peak of energy whereas the *time average intensity* is the average intensity calculated over the time between pulses.

Summary

An understanding of basic ultrasound physics is required to enable the physician to understand how images are produced. It enables an understanding of why artefacts happen and enables the physician to appreciate the limitations of ultrasound and how to manipulate the machine to improve images. This will be covered in the following chapter.

References

1 AIUM. Bio-effect considerations for the safety of diagnostic ultrasound. *J Ultrasound Medicine* 1988;**7** (Suppl 9): s1–s38.

Further reading

McDicken WN. *Diagnostic Ultrasonics, 4th edn.* Philadelphia: WB Saunders, 1997.

Meire HB, Cosgrove DO, Dewbury KC, Farrant P. *Clinical Ultrasound: A Comprehensive Text – Abdominal and General Ultrasound, 2nd edn.* Philadelphia: WB Saunders, 2001.

Rumack CM, Wilson SR, Charboneau JW. *Diagnostic Ultrasound, 2nd edn.* Philadelphia: Mosby, 1998.

3 Image acquisition and artefacts

OTTO CHAN

Objectives
- To learn how to turn ultrasound machines on and off
- To understand what are the key functions available and how to optimise image acquisition
- To understand what all the knobs do and where to find them on the control panel
- To understand and recognise basic US artefacts

Introduction

It is only in the past 5–10 years that clinicians have realised the value of ultrasound (US). Unfortunately, there is limited access to good US training for clinicians so clinicians have started buying and using US machines without appropriate training. This chapter is specifically dedicated to helping the clinician, in how to get started on a US machine for the first time and how to recognise basic artefacts. Therefore, by definition, there will be a significant amount of overlap in the topics covered in this chapter and Chapter 2. It is not within the scope of this chapter to explain the physics and readers are advised to cross reference with Chapter 2.

US machines are in effect made up of three basic components: the monitor, the computer and the probes (Figure 3.1). There are very basic US machines, which are much smaller in size and are truly portable or even handheld with a rechargeable battery (Figure 3.2). There is a range of much larger and more complex US machines, which obviously are more expensive and the level of expertise necessary to use these is much greater. Unfortunately, the different US machines available makes the choice of which one to purchase bewildering and the cost can vary from £10 000 for a handheld US machine with two probes to over £200 000 for an US machine with all the extras.

The manufacturers have come up with a huge range of options and extras; many of these are not necessary for basic imaging. The problem for most clinicians, who encounter a US machine for the first time, is that there is no standardised control panel. Most machines use either a mixture of keys, levers (paddle controls), knobs, push buttons,

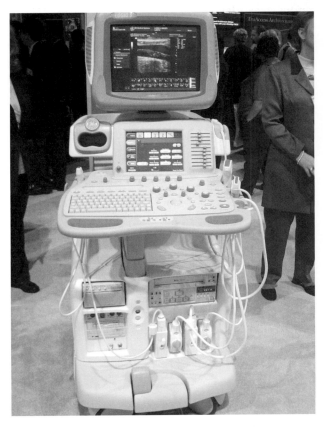

Figure 3.1 The basic components of an ultrasound machine are the monitor, the computer, and the probes.

dials, spin controls, slide controls, or a screen menu to select options and to change different parameters and functions, so for the sake of simplicity, these will all be referred to as knobs (hence knobology). The knobs are usually labelled; unfortunately, the name given for individual functions is not standardised and often there is only either an initial or a symbol. Some new US machines only use symbols and have no labelling, in order to save space (Figure 3.3). Therefore, prior to using the US machine for the first time, it is essential to familiarise oneself with the standard functions available and how to use them.

This chapter will attempt to provide a list of all the key functions, the name or symbol given in order to recognise the knob, and the position of the knob on the control panel on most machines. The top of the range US machines usually duplicate the functions by providing a screen

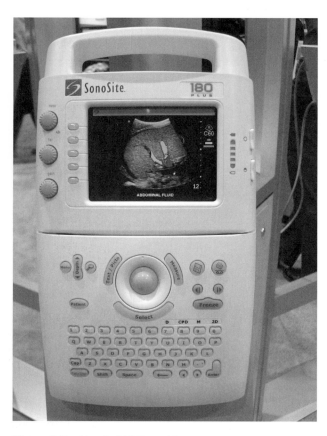

Figure 3.2 Handheld US machine.

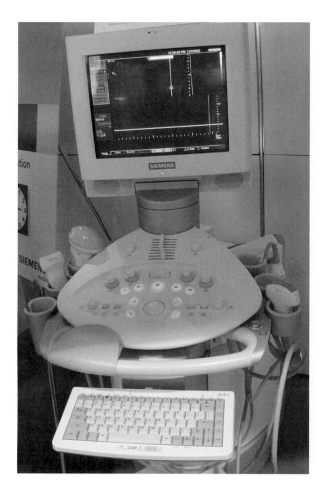

Figure 3.4 Slimline US machine.

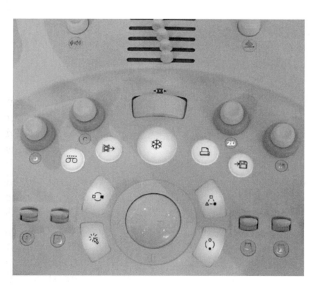

Figure 3.3 Symbols on an US machine.

menu or preset key function knobs, which can be preset either by the manufacturer or tailor-made for the individual clinician. This can save a huge amount of time later, in particular in relation to labelling images, as most practitioners usually have their own set routine on how to scan and how to label individual images.

Whilst there is a huge variation in the design and layout of the main control panel, there are some general rules, which most manufacturers and US machines follow. Within the range of basic to top of the range US machines, each manufacturer has a relatively similar layout. The main key functions are generally at the front, on the centre or just to the right of the midline and most of these functions are within easy reach (that is, a hand's breadth) and usually surround the tracker ball. All the remaining key functions tend to be grouped together around the main key functions (for example Doppler functions) on the control panel.

The keyboard is usually right above the main key function knobs or at the top of the control panel. However, some of the portable US machines and some of the new slimline US machines have a keyboard that slides out from under the main key function knobs and under the control panel (Figure 3.4).

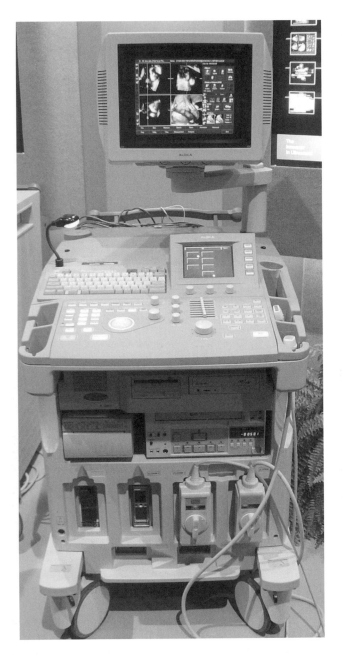

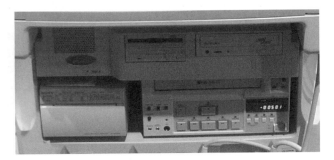

Figure 3.5 Modern US machines have a large range of extras.

How to get started

There is a huge range of US machines and these vary from simple portable units to top of the range machines which usually have many extras, including a black and white and/or colour printer, a video, a CD or DVD recorder, a zip drive and a foot switch (Figure 3.5). These items may all need a separate power supply or may be incorporated onto the main computer.

The most basic US machines, which are portable and may have a portable battery, usually have only one on/off switch for the monitor and the computer together. It is important not to forget to charge the battery before using it.

The US machine is in effect a computer with a monitor, and just like any home computer it must be turned off properly, in order for it to function correctly when turned on the next time. The US machine therefore has a mains lead to plug onto the wall and often has an independent switch at the back to provide a power supply to the US machine as a whole. Once the power supply is turned on, the US machine has a separate switch to turn on the computer and the monitor; this is usually either on the left side of the machine, on the side or on the top left side of the main control panel.

It normally takes a few minutes for the computer to turn on and log on, just like a home computer. Therefore, if there is an emergency, for example focused assessment with sonography for trauma (FAST), the US machine should be turned on early, in order to avoid delay.

Prior to scanning, the patient's name and hospital number should be typed in. Identify the knob, which should be on the top left hand side of the screen (Patient/Patient, ID/Patient, Status/Patient, Data/New Patient) and enter all the relevant details. Once the patient data has been entered, the main menu will be displayed on the monitor.

The first option before scanning will be to select which transducer to use. Most basic portable US units will only have one transducer, and if a different transducer is going to be used the transducer has to be changed. However, the larger machines usually have several ports for at least 2–4 transducers and often have different types of ports for different transducers (Figure 3.6). The ports are usually at the bottom of the machine facing your feet or on the right side of the machine, near the front. Simply pick up the plug attached and follow the lead to the correct probe.

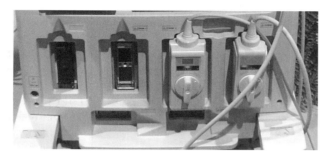

Figure 3.6 Ports for transducers.

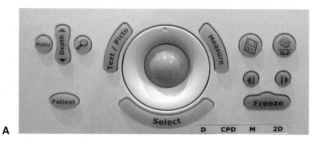

A

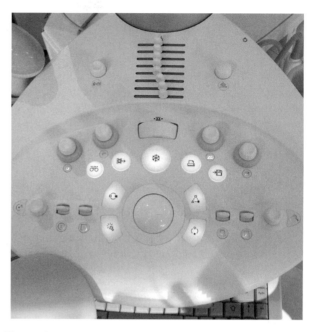

Figure 3.8 Control panel using all knobs.

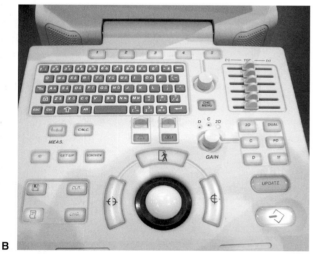

B

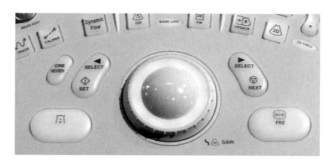

Figure 3.9 Key function controls – this includes the controls that are most commonly used, in particular the tracker ball, freeze, set and print buttons.

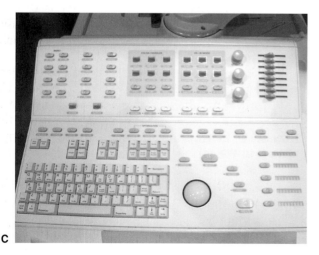

C

Figure 3.7 Different layouts of control panels.

The screen will give you a list of the probes plugged in and the options available. Once the correct probe has been selected, the screen will ask for a body part to be selected. It is important to select the correct body part, as the manufacturers have preset the probe for a particular area and set the appropriate Doppler flow characteristics for that body part. It is not uncommon to find a trainee using a high frequency probe to examine testes with "abdomen" selected as the body part. Not surprisingly, the settings are unlikely to provide for optimal scanning.

Once the body part has been selected, the US machine is ready for scanning and the correct parameters will need to be adjusted for each individual patient and often for each individual image. It is important not to forget that the

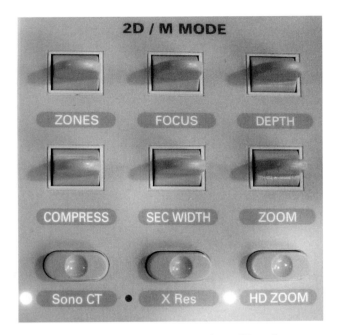

Figure 3.10   Image controls – this adjusts 2D real time grey-scale imaging.

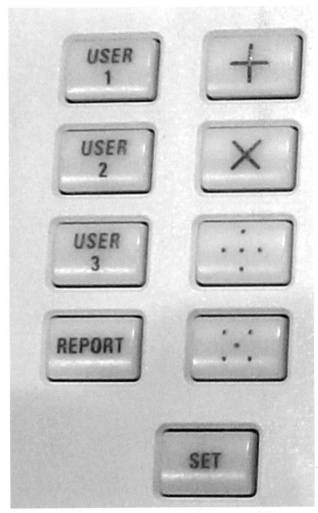

Figure 3.11   Measurement controls – these knobs are used in conjunction with the tracker ball to measure and annotate.

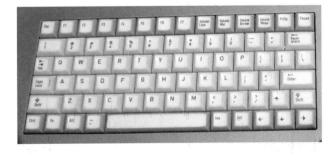

Figure 3.12   Keyboard – standardised keyboard with an additional array of text and control keys.

manufacturers set the US machine for the "perfect" patient and that a large proportion of patients are either too fat or too thin.

Control panel

Different manufacturers have different layouts to the main control panel (Figures 3.7a, 3.7b and 3.7c). However, there is a huge variation, even between different US machines, in where each knob is located and what each knob is called. In addition, even on any one machine, the control used to select a particular parameter may be a push button, knob, dial, paddle control (lever), spin or slide control (Figure 3.8). Therefore, as previously discussed, for the sake of simplicity, all these controls will be referred to generally as knobs (hence knobology).

In general, the control panel is arranged into layout groups, which enhance operator interaction. Not infrequently, for a single function, several controls are necessary and therefore these function knobs are grouped together.

Function groups

The function groups are illustrated in figures 3.9 to 3.16.

Knobology

This section will attempt to explain what each knob does, where to locate it, and, where relevant, how to adjust it for optimal scanning. It is

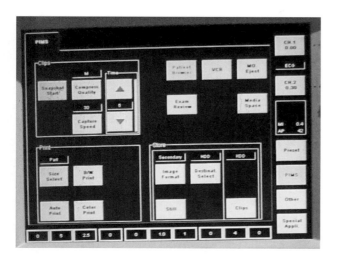

Figure 3.13 Touch panel display – sometimes it is part of the monitor and occasionally it is part of the main control panel. It duplicates many of the other functions and replaces many knobs.

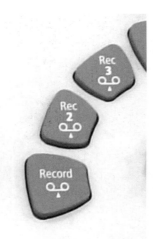

Figure 3.15 Peripheral controls – this relates to additional devices such as video, colour printer, optical disc storage, network imaging, or a paper printer.

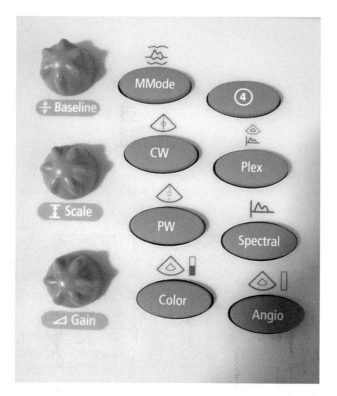

Figure 3.14 Doppler controls – this group of controls relates purely to Doppler function controls.

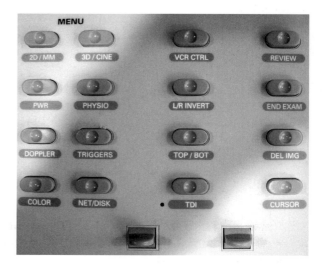

Figure 3.16 Special function keys – this includes the preset functions, dual display function, invert image, and other specialised functions such as extended field of view scanning (for example Siescape).

Patient/patient, ID/patient, status/patient, data/new patient (Figure 3.17)

This knob is usually a push button and often only has a symbol. It is usually found on the left side, right at the back of the control panel or on the keyboard. It is essential that prior to scanning, all the patient details are entered, including the hospital number, if images are going to be recorded. On portable and emergency US scans, it may be quicker sometimes to scan, image and print and then to hand write the name and then date and sign the scan at the back of the paper print.

important to refer to the individual manufacturer's manual for a more detailed account of each key function, where to find it on the control panel, and how to preset functions before scanning.

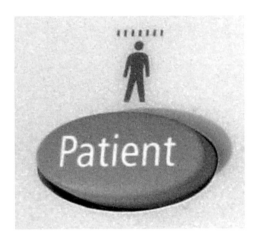

Figure 3.17   Patient button.

Probe/scan, head/transducers (Figure 3.18)

There are numerous US transducers (probes) available on the market, but on each individual US machine there is usually only a limited selection. Which US transducers to use depends predominantly on which organ is being examined.

The higher the frequency, the better the resolution (and therefore the better the image), but unfortunately, as the frequency increases, so the penetration is reduced. Therefore, as a general rule, the highest frequency transducers should be used, in order to obtain an image:

- high frequency transducers (7·5 MHz to over 12 MHz) – suitable for superficial structures, such as thyroid, breast, testes and salivary glands
- medium frequency transducers (5 MHz) – suitable for paediatric abdominal US and thin adult patients
- low frequency transducers (2·5 MHz to 3·5 MHz) – used for general adult abdominal and pelvic US.

Transducers are also classified by the shape of the beam. The choice of the shape of the transducer is predominantly dependent on the footprint (that is, the area of contact with the patient).

- Sector scanners (Figure 3.18a) – these have a small footprint and produce a fan-shaped image. They are usually very good for imaging organs with poor access, such as neonatal heads, intercostals, abdominal scanning and cardiac scanning.

- Linear scanners (Figure 3.18b) – they produce a rectangular image and are very popular for high frequency superficial scanning, in particular musculoskeletal imaging.
- Curvilinear scanners (Figure 3.18c) – these transducers combine a large footprint with the advantages of the sector scanner.
- Annular array scanners (Figure 3.18d) – these scanners produce a circular image and are used mainly for transrectal and transvaginal scanning. There are also other more specialised probes for endoscopic and intravascular imaging.

Phased array transducers produce a sector scan by steering the beam electronically and have the advantage of no moving parts compared to mechanical transducers. Different types of extended field of view scanning have partly overcome the disadvantage of small footprint scanners. This allows the array transducers to be moved along and an extended image obtained (for example Siescape in Siemens US machines).

Tracker ball (Figure 3.19)

The tracker ball is one of the only constant features of US machine keyboards. It is in effect the equivalent of the mouse on a home computer and is used for virtually all functions. It can:

- move the cursor on the monitor
- move the cursor between patient data
- be used for measurement of calliper control points
- create text and arrow annotations
- be used with Doppler, to position sample and range gate.

In addition, on some US machines it also acts as the replay knob for the cine loop facility, a very useful accessory for uncooperative patients and in paediatric US. Therefore, it is usually surrounded by the main key function knobs, in particular the freeze, set, measure and print knobs.

Freeze (Figure 3.19)

The frame freeze knob halts real time (live) imaging and allows a single image to be viewed

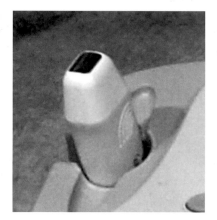

A

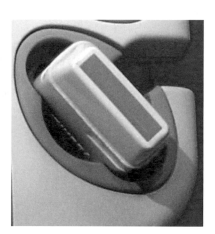

B

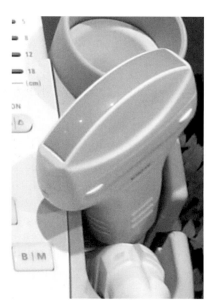

C

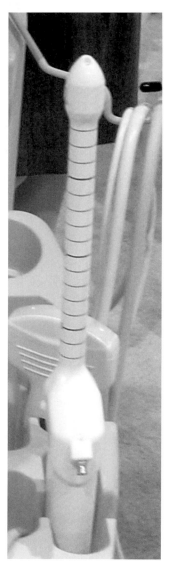

D

Figure 3.18 Probes. (**A**) Sector scanner. (**B**) Linear Scanner. (**C**) Curvilinear scanner. (**D**) Annular array scanner.

by stopping new echo values overwriting those already stored. This allows acquisition of images and static measurements taken with the callipers. Unfreezing the image allows overwriting of previously stored data and therefore continuing real time scanning.

Most transducers have a dimple or bump at one end to allow orientation of the transducer to the screen. By convention this marker represents the left side of the screen when the operator looks at it. In transverse imaging the marker should be oriented to the patient's right and in longitudinal section to the head. It is wise to check this by touching the end of the probe and looking at the

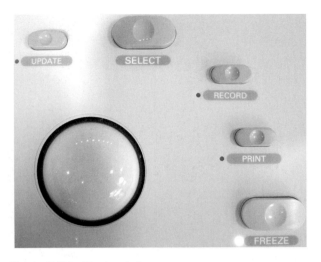

Figure 3.19   Tracker ball.

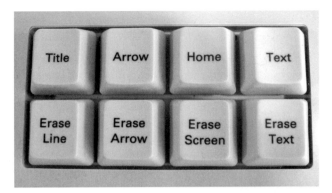

Figure 3.20   Preset labels.

location of the reflections on the screen each time the transducer is picked up.

Select/set (Figure 3.19)

The set knob is usually a push button right next to the tracker ball. The set and tracker ball are invariably used together and therefore all the functions of the tracker ball are related to the set knob.

The select button in effect is the equivalent of double clicking the mouse on a home computer and enables selection of a menu on the monitor.

Label/ABC/text/home (Figure 3.20)

This knob is usually a push button near the keyboard. This knob brings a cursor onto the screen, which allows text to be typed within the image. The position of where to place the text is selected using the tracker ball. The home knob will localise the text position to a specific site.

A huge amount of time is spent on labelling images, which are rarely reviewed as US is a very subjective imaging modality. Therefore, only images that cannot be recognised should be labelled fully.

Preset labels/preset/text A, B, C and D (Figure 3.20)

Where extensive labelling is required or practised, it is advisable to have preset labelling, which is individualised and therefore at a touch of the knob; specific labelling is performed in a predictable sequence.

Erase line/erase text/erase screen (Figure 3.20)

The erase knobs in general are push buttons or part of the keyboard. These knobs can selectively delete either line by line or all the text typed on the screen.

Depth

The depth control of most US machines is done using paddle controls (levers). The correct depth of imaging should be selected, otherwise the image is extremely small and the better resolution is lost. In addition, if a large area is sampled, there will be an increase in the noise seen, thus also degrading the image further.

In general, reducing depth is a very efficient way of improving the quality of the image. On the top of the range US machines, the multi-frequency probes actually image the more superficial structures at a higher frequency compared to the deeper structures; once again this will significantly improve imaging.

Time or depth gain compensation (TGC or DGC) (Figure 3.21)

The TGC can be easily identified as a set of slide controls. On small portable US machines, it can be a simple near and far gain two switch but on virtually all other models it is a complex series of 6–10 slide controls, which individually control the gain at a particular depth.

As the US beam progresses through the tissues, the beam inherently loses power. This is compensated for automatically in the US machine by the TGC/DGC. The amount of automatic

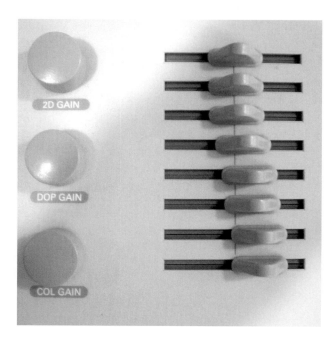

Figure 3.21   Time gain compensation.

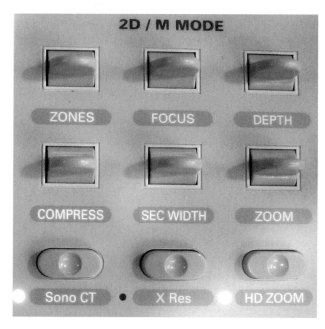

Figure 3.22   Focus and magnification.

compensation is determined by the organ and probe selected at the start of the US scan and the manufacturers decide on the amount of compensation, based on expected tissue attenuation coefficients. If the tissues being imaged are higher than expected, then the appropriate adjustments need to be made to make the image brighter, by sliding the slide controls to the right. The converse is that if the tissues have a tissue attenuation coefficient less than expected, then the image will be brighter and therefore the TGC needs to be adjusted by pushing the series of slide controls to the left.

The top of the range US machines have automated TGC and gain controls. This can be very helpful for difficult patients and also trainees who have just started scanning and are unsure of what parameters to use.

Gain (Figure 3.21)

The gain control is usually a dial, or part of or around the tracker ball, and controls the overall gain without the ability to control the gain at different depths like the TGC. The gain and TGC should be used together, to provide a relatively even image. However, the decision of whether to scan bright or dark is very much a personal one and US is extremely subjective.

On the whole and as a generalisation, most experienced practitioners tend to scan darker than the trainee and the mistakes tend to be made when scanning too bright. Subtle changes in echogenicity tend to be more readily detected with darker imaging.

Focus (Figure 3.22)

The focus control is usually a paddle control next to the depth and zoom controls. The physics and theoretical methods for focusing an US beam are quite complex. In effect, it is extremely important to get the focus at the depth of interest. In doing so, the beam thickness is reduced in the focal region, which directly improves both the contrast and spatial resolution.

Sometimes, the image can be significantly improved by having the focus set at more than one level. The more levels of focus, the slower the frame rate, which makes imaging quite tiring and makes real-time imaging of moving structures very awkward and tiring.

Magnification (Figure 3.22)

The magnification control is a paddle control next to all the other image controls. Magnification can usually be done before or after freezing an image and can therefore be a post-processing control. The knob magnifies the entire image and the image size on the screen. The disadvantage is that it does not improve contrast or spatial resolution and the image becomes more grainy. One of the main advantages is that measurements can be made more accurately by magnifying the image.

Zoom/HD zoom (Figure 3.22)

The zoom control is a paddle or push button control next to all the other image controls. This usually needs to be done with the tracker ball, to select the size of the sample and the position of the sampling area.

This function is similar to magnification, except that the sample size is smaller and therefore there is no degradation of the image, despite a larger screen. With high definition zoom, the sample size is smaller, there is a reduction on sample width leading to a faster frame rate and improvement of the spatial and contrast resolution, and reduction in movement artefact.

Measure/callipers

This knob is usually next to the tracker ball and is usually a push button. When selected, the cursor points appear. There are numerous parameters that can be used for measurement on different US machines. However, the vast proportion of measurements are linear. Most US machines use the tracker ball and a calliper system. There are numerous systems, which move the calliper spot back to the midline or there are several knobs on some US machines for separate measurements – these are extremely cumbersome and annoying. The simplest method is one knob for the callipers, movement with the tracker ball, and using the set knob to obtain the measurement. To obtain a second set of callipers, the knob is pressed again and a different set of callipers appears. This facility can then be repeated as many times as necessary and gets over the problem of too many knobs on the main keyboard.

In general, only linear measurements are necessary. Rarely, in particular in obstetrics scanning, more complex shapes need to be measured and this facility is available on most US machines.

Print

In radiology departments over the next decade, most of the US images will be recorded on the

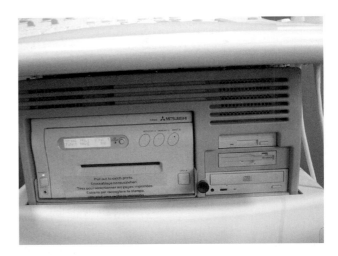

Figure 3.23 Inbuilt storage facility linked to floppy disk, CD and DVD drive.

main digitised (PACS) system. However, at present most US machines are linked onto a laser printer in US departments.

In many US departments, there is at least one US machine with a colour printer, predominantly for printing colour Doppler images. Invariably, the colour printer is not part of the US machine but a stand alone unit.

Most portable US machines have either no printer facility or only a paper printer and in many ways, that is all that is necessary at present. However, as more clinicians practise US, it is clear that paper print records as the sole means of keeping a record are not satisfactory. Many of the newer portable US machines, and certainly most medium and top of the range machines, have an in-built image storage facility and most can be linked to either a floppy disk, CD, DVD, zip drive, or video machine (Figure 3.23).

Cine (Figure 3.24)

The cine facility is inbuilt into the US memory and frame freeze facility on most medium and top of the range US machines. When the frame freeze knob is pressed, a single frame is seen on the monitor. However, the computer records several seconds of imaging prior to the freeze facility. These images can be viewed frame by frame by using the cine knob (usually a dial, either incorporated into the tracker ball or next to the freeze knob).

The facility is extremely helpful in uncooperative patients, portable US, paediatric scanning and in patients who cannot follow instructions.

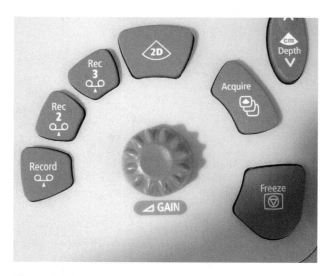

Figure 3.24   Cine, image store, and video recording facilities.

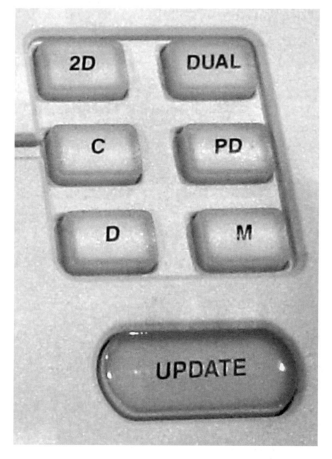

Image store (Figure 3.24)

The image store is the equivalent to the hard disk on a home computer and allows storage of data, which is obviously limited by the size of the memory. Most US machines with this facility have some form of recording device, either a floppy drive, CD, or DVD.

Figure 3.25   Doppler imaging.

Video (Figure 3.24)

Video recording facilities are not necessary except in obstetric and cardiac scanning. It is however a very useful facility to have available for training purposes or to record a difficult case, when more senior assistance is not available at the time of the examination.

Doppler (Figure 3.25)

The basic principles of Doppler US have been covered in other chapters and are not within the scope of this chapter. Recent advances and clinical acceptance of Doppler US has made it almost an essential component of any US machine. It is almost certain that in the next few years colour Doppler will be available on even the most basic portable US machines as new guidelines for best clinical practice will insist on US being used for vascular access and all forms of intervention being done under image guidance.

- *2D mode* – this returns the scanner to real time grey scale imaging.
- *M-mode* – this displays M-mode imaging.
- *C-mode* – this displays colour Doppler imaging.
- *Power* – this displays power Doppler imaging.
- Dual image – this allows two images to be displayed on the monitor, side-by-side. One image can be scanned live, then the image needs to be frozen before the other image can be activated.
- Next image/L/R or symbol – this is used in conjunction with the dual image and selects which image is active and can be viewed in real time.
- Image invert/L/R/top/bottom – this selects the left/right orientation of the 2D image. In effect, it has the same result as turning the probe round 180 degrees. It is very helpful to have this function when the transducer has an asymmetrical shape (jockey stick high resolution probe), allowing better contact and access for scanning.

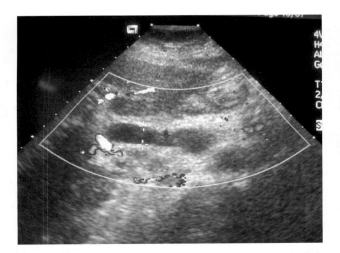

Figure 3.26 Acoustic shadowing.

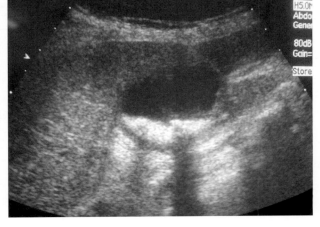

Figure 3.27 Edge shadows.

Artefacts

The true definition of an artefact in radiology is any image that doesn't exist and is man-made. Therefore, in radiology, most of the time, artefacts are unwanted and cause degradation of imaging. US is very prone to artefacts, but unlike other imaging modalities, in US many artefacts are diagnostically very useful. Therefore, it is essential that clinicians are fully aware of and can recognise artefacts, in order to avoid diagnostic errors.

Acoustic shadowing (Figure 3.26)

This appears as a very dark area directly behind a very echogenic area and is due to complete absorption or reflection of the US beam. The tissue it hits is of a much higher attenuation coefficient than the surrounding tissues and therefore the TGC provides an inaccurate correction, leading to the shadow or distal shadow. Acoustic shadows are therefore produced by highly reflective structures, such as calcification, bone, metal, gas bubbles, and stones.

Edge shadows are seen when a cystic structure casts a very narrow acoustic shadow from the edge (Figure 3.27). The exact explanation is still debated, but it is a regular artefact seen around cystic structures.

Acoustic enhancement (Figure 3.28)

This in effect is the reverse of acoustic shadowing, where the US beam goes through an area where the tissues attenuate less than the

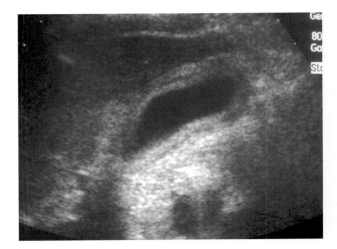

Figure 3.28 Acoustic enhancement.

surrounding tissues and therefore there is a very bright area behind the structure, again due to inaccurate correction by the DGC. Acoustic enhancement is seen behind all cystic structures, such as the gall bladder and bladder, and behind cystic collections and most abscesses.

Mirror artefact (Figure 3.29)

It is assumed that a US beam returns directly to the transducer after one reflection. However, if there are multiple reflections, then there is the possibility of multiple images being produced. Since the path of these images is longer than the original image, the corresponding images are seen lying deeper.

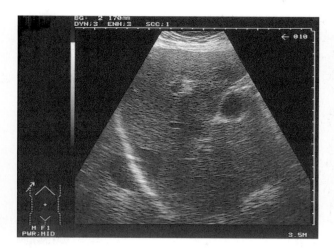

Figure 3.29 Mirror artefact.

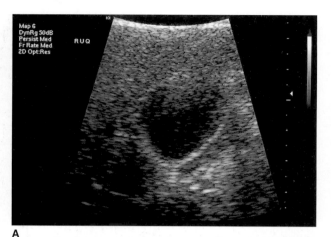

A

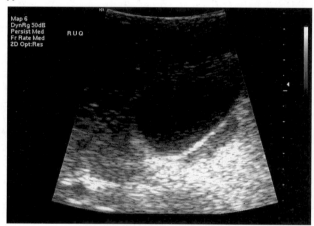

B

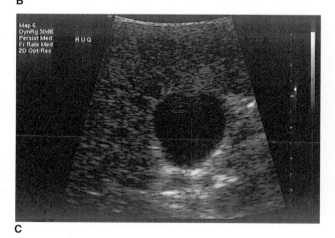

C

Figure 3.30 Reverberation.

A single echo will lead to an image lying immediately deep to the original image, usually on the opposite side of a sharply reflective surface and equidistant from it. A typical mirror image is seen on either side of the diaphragm.

Reverberation (Figure 3.30)

The same principles are used to explain reverberation artefacts, except that these are made from multiple repeat echoes from parallel, highly reflective structures. A striped pattern results over the surface of an organ when in close proximity to the skin.

Comet tail or ring down artefact (Figure 3.31)

A striped pattern in a bright streak called a comet tail is sometimes seen in highly reflective structures such as clips, catheters, implants, and foreign bodies.

Noise (Figure 3.32)

Noise is unfortunately seen in all types of imaging and almost invariably represents unwanted artefact. Excess amplification, random voltage changes at low levels, and random vibration of molecules can all cause random noise.

Structured noise can occur from body or probe movement; this does not really affect grey scale imaging but has some effect on Doppler motion artefacts.

Beam width and orthogonal width artefacts

The true US beam is not actually uniform and in particular the edges are not sharply defined; the

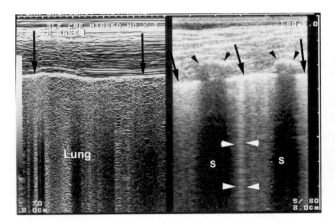

Figure 3.31   Comet tail.

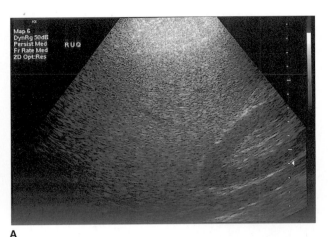

A

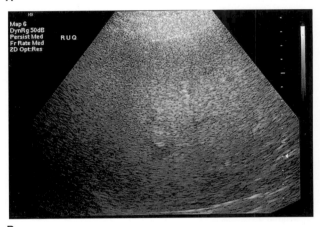

B

Figure 3.32   Noise can be caused by excess amplification, random low level voltage changes, and random vibration of molecules.

beam is concentrated centrally and falls progressively from the centre. This leads to beam width artefacts and orthogonal beam width artefacts.

Summary

This chapter is no more than an introduction and a summary of the user information, getting started, control panel, and 2D imaging chapters in the reference manual of most US machines. An attempt has been made to make some sense of the overall layout of US machines, from the most basic to the top of the range. In addition, a further attempt has been made to explain what all the knobs do and how to use them.

However, it is in no way supposed to replace the reference manual of any individual machine, and the information in this chapter is in many ways the minimum necessary before one first starts scanning.

The artefacts section is no more than a summary of the common artefacts seen in routine scanning and ones that one should at least recognise, in order to avoid basic and embarrassing errors, which should be easily avoidable.

4 Focussed assessment with sonography for trauma (FAST)

ADAM BROOKS, M GAGE OSCHNER

Objectives
- To assess the role of FAST in the investigation of abdominal trauma
- To define the principles of FAST
- To review the practical technique for FAST
- To present a FAST trauma algorithm

Introduction

Over the last ten years Focussed Assessment with Sonography for Trauma (FAST) has become the standard resuscitation room investigation for the evaluation of the trauma patient throughout Europe and North America. The technique is gradually being accepted in emergency departments (EDs) in the United Kingdom, Australia and internationally and with the development of sophisticated handheld ultrasound systems the value of this rapid and accurate technique is becoming apparent in the military and pre-hospital environment. Numerous studies have repeatedly shown that FAST is valuable in the assessment of blunt abdominal trauma in the emergency room, especially in the unstable multiply injured patient.

The introduction of FAST has at times been contentious, when surgeons and physicians have taken up the technology. The development of any new technology and its introduction to a clinical environment must be undertaken with control and care and the limitations of the technique and adequate training of personnel need to be addressed.

The development of FAST

Ultrasound has been used for the investigation and treatment of medical conditions since the 1950s. However it was not until the 1970s that it was first used in the assessment of the injured patient. Kristensen's report in 1971 on the use of US for the diagnosis of splenic haematomas was rapidly followed by further case reports on the detection of liver injuries and renal haematomas by US. The initial enthusiasm continued with prospective work that initially concentrated on the detection of organ injury and sensitivities up to 80% were reported for the detection of splenic injury. The inclusion of attempts to define organ injury as well as intraperitoneal bleeding reduced the sensitivity of these early reports and it rapidly became clear that haemoperitoneum could be detected more reliably than specific organ injury.

From here the technique developed rapidly with the focus firmly on the detection of intra-abdominal bleeding. Grace Rozycki, from the USA, assessed the ability of surgeons (non-radiologists) to use the technique for the evaluation of the trauma patient in the emergency room. The ability of non-radiologists to perform trauma US reliably was clearly defined in studies published by her group in 1993 and 1995 and the acronym FAST, 'Focused Abdominal Sonogram for Trauma', was introduced. FAST rapidly developed to regions beyond the abdomen and in recognition of this the term 'Focused Assessment with Sonography for Trauma' was accepted at the International Consensus Conference in 1997.

Investigation of abdominal trauma

It has been widely recognised for many years that the abdominal evaluation of the trauma patient is unreliable; hampered by head injury, alcohol, or recreational drugs. Even in the hands of experts the physical examination is little better than guesswork. An alternative technique has been sought that could provide the frontline emergency physicians and surgeons with rapid, sensitive, and accurate information on abdominal injuries at the bedside. To date no single modality meets these criteria. The current alternative techniques are reviewed in brief.

Diagnostic peritoneal lavage (DPL)

Following the original description of the technique in 1965, for many years DPL was considered the gold standard for the investigation of blunt abdominal trauma. Despite advances in technology and imaging many institutions continue to use it as the primary bedside investigation.

The open and closed percutaneous techniques have been shown to have equal sensitivity and using lavage cell counts of 100 000 red cells per mm³ (RCC) and 500 white cells per mm³ the technique provides reliable and reproducible results in blunt trauma with a sensitivity of 90% and accuracy of 97% for intraperitoneal bleeding. These values provide an appropriate balance between sensitivity and non-therapeutic laparotomy that may approach 10–15%. Unfortunately some lavage results remain equivocal (RCC 50 000 – 100 000) and must be interpreted with caution. Repeated clinical assessment and alternative investigations such as CT in stable patients are required to augment decision making in this group. DPL is far less valuable in penetrating injury, rather like FAST. A positive lavage is a strong predictor of injury; however the small amounts of blood that may be associated with isolated puncture wounds reduce the sensitivity and lavage counts between 1000 and 10 000 red cells per mm³ are used to counter this.

DPL is an invasive technique and a small incidence of iatrogenic injuries have been reported. There are a number of relative contraindications to DPL including obesity, pregnancy, and multiple abdominal scars.

Computerised tomography (CT)

The contrast enhanced helical CT scan is the investigation of choice in the cardiovascularly stable trauma patient. A full trauma series with 1 cm cuts from the top of the diaphragm to the pubic symphysis can be obtained within minutes with modern scanners.

CT imaging provides organ specificity in abdominal trauma and allows imaging of the retroperitoneal structures. The images can be used to grade both the severity of organ injury and the degree of haemoperitoneum, both of which have been shown to be valuable predictors for the success of non-operative management. In the evaluation of abdominal injury CT has a reported sensitivity of 88% and a negative predictive value of 97%. The accuracy of CT in the evaluation of small intestine and pancreatic injuries has been questioned.

CT scanners are often located at a distance from the ED and monitoring difficulties during the scan mean that CT is not appropriate for the unstable patient.

Diagnostic laparoscopy (DL)

In blunt abdominal trauma laparoscopy does not improve outcome compared to DPL. It is time consuming, resource intensive and expensive. The technique can be limited by the presence of significant volumes of blood and there is limited ability to assess the small bowel and retroperitoneum.

Laparoscopy is valuable in the assessment of suspected diaphragm rupture in stable patients and in the evaluation of peritoneal penetration in abdominal and thoraco-abdominal stab wounds.

Focussed assessment with sonography for trauma (FAST)

Since the introduction of FAST in the early 1990s numerous papers have been published that validate the technique and confirm its value in the evaluation of abdominal trauma. The largest series to date, of over 2500 patients, reported a sensitivity of 86%, specificity of 98%, and accuracy of 97% for the detection of intra-abdominal injuries in blunt trauma. Although early results of trauma ultrasound were slightly disappointing, the adoption of the FAST principles advocated by Rozycki et al and the end point of the investigation being accepted as the detection of haemoperitoneum, rather than organ injury, has led to improvements and excellent values being reported. Numerous papers have now been published detailing sensitivity ranging from 81–88·2% for FAST with specificity of 90–99·7% (see Table 4.1).

FAST has been compared against CT, DPL, and laparoscopy in several papers in the investigation of blunt abdominal trauma. Table 4.2 summarises and compares the published sensitivity and specificity of these modalities. These papers have shown that FAST is accurate, rapid, and less expensive than the alternatives. However no single investigation is appropriate for the investigation of abdominal trauma in every situation and these modalities should be viewed as being complementary.

Table 4.1 Comparison of values for sensitivity and specificity of FAST

	Year	Patients	Sensitivity %	Specificity %
Dolich	2001	2576	86	90
Healey	1996	745	88·2	97·7
McKenney	1996	1000	88	99
Rozycki	1995	371	81·5	99·7
Boulanger	1995	206	81	98

Table 4.2 Comparison of diagnostic tools for abdominal trauma

	Sensitivity %	Specificity %
DPL	95	99
Computer Tomography	88	98
Ultrasound	79–88·2	90–99·7

Table 4.3 Comparison of use of FAST by radiologists and non-radiologists

	Rozycki		Buzzas	
	NR	R	NR	R
Sensitivity	93·4%	90·8%	79·5%	79·5%
Specificity	98·7%	99·2%	97·5%	99·3%
Accuracy	97·5%	97·8%		

NR, Non-radiologists; R, Radiologists

FAST has a number of advantages. It is non-invasive, easily repeatable, and modern hand carried systems have now been validated in trauma. Critics highlight the technical limitations of ultrasound. These are discussed below together with the operator-dependent nature of the investigation; however with appropriate training and the FAST technique this appears less of an issue.

Radiologist v non-radiologist

The introduction of trauma ultrasound in the emergency room has, at times, brought emergency physicians and surgeons into direct confrontation with radiologists. As a result there have been a number of difficulties with the introduction of this technique in centres around the world. To address the perceived issues of non-radiologists with limited training performing trauma ultrasound Rozycki compared a series of papers describing non-radiologist FAST examination with trauma ultrasound performed by a radiologist. The results from this analysis revealed that in terms of sensitivity, specificity, and accuracy for detecting haemoperitoneum, non radiologists compared favourably with the radiologists (Table 4.3). This has since been confirmed in a prospective study from the USA, which showed no significant difference in sensitivity or specificity between surgeons/physicians and radiologists performing FAST.

FAST in penetrating abdominal trauma

Although the investigation of choice in the immediate evaluation of blunt abdominal trauma, the application of FAST in penetrating injury remains contentious. The limited volume of blood associated with some penetrating injuries may be missed by FAST and has reduced the sensitivity of the technique to only 42% in some series. If FAST is used as the initial investigation of trauma patients with penetrating injuries then a positive FAST is a strong predictor of significant injury. Additional investigations to exclude occult injury are essential if FAST is negative.

Attempts have been made to use high frequency ultrasound to evaluate penetrating wound tracts for pleural or peritoneal breach. This technique has not been widely accepted.

The FAST technique

Basics

FAST should be undertaken using a 3–5 MHz transducer of appropriate dimensions such that it can be orientated in the rib spaces. The probe should be held predominantly in the saggital plane to allow easier orientation and recognition of the anatomy.

The basis of FAST is the detection of blood in any of the three dependent regions of the abdomen where blood tends to collect: perihepatic space,

perisplenic space, or pelvis. In addition a view of
the pericardium is studied to look for evidence of
cardiac tamponade. These four ultrasound windows
are known as the four Ps.

Pericardial area

The subxiphoid pericardial view looks for
blood in the pericardial sac and tamponade.

Probe position

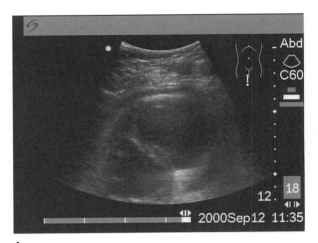

A

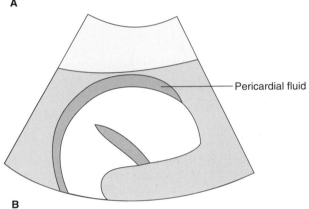

B

Figure 4.2 Pericardial effusion.

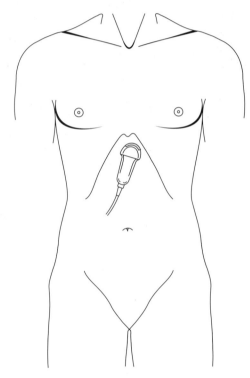

Figure 4.1 Pericardial probe position. Position the
transducer just below the xiphoid process. The probe is then
rotated cephalad and slightly toward the left shoulder with
firm downward pressure until a satisfactory picture of the
heart and pericardial space is obtained.

Patient Although frequently the patient will be
unable to cooperate a deep inspiration may
improve the image by bringing the mediastinal
structures downwards.

Images The liver is used as a window through
which to view the heart. A pericardial effusion
is recognised as an anechoic or dark stripe
between the (moving) ventricular wall and the
pericardium (see Figures 4.2 and 4.3).

Points and pitfalls

- The image must be closely scrutinised to
  ensure that the heart border and pericardium
  are clearly identified.
- Clotted blood in the pericardium may not be as
  obvious as unclotted blood as the contrast
  between ventricle and blood is reduced. This
  could lead to a false negative result.
- Occasionally an adequate view of the
  pericardial space through the subxiphoid
  position is technically impossible due to
  obesity or pain. In this situation the transducer
  can be oriented transversely in the left third or
  fourth intercostal space a few centimetres
  lateral to the sternum.

Perihepatic

Fluid collects either between the liver and
diaphragm or in the hepatorenal space (Rutherford
Morison's Pouch).

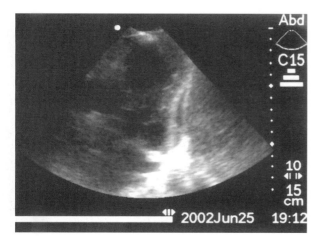

A

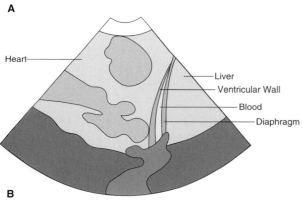

B

Figure 4.3　Pericardial view. (**A**) Positive image. (**B**) Drawing.

Probe position

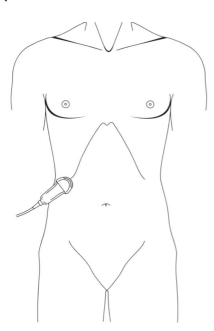

Figure 4.4　Perihepatic probe position. Locate the transducer in the anterior axillary line in approximately the tenth intercostal space. The image obtained should reveal the liver and right kidney and fluid should be looked for at the interface between the two organs.

Patient　In acute trauma the patient is nearly always scanned supine with the doctor on the patient's right. To optimise the perihepatic image a deep breath by the patient may bring the structures down into view.

Images

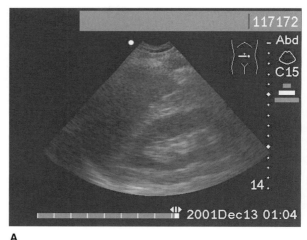

A

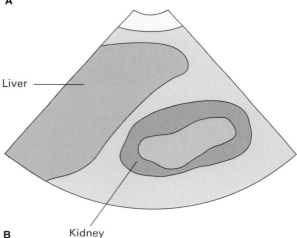

B　Kidney

Figure 4.5　Perihepatic view. (**A**) Normal image (**B**) Drawing.

Points and pitfalls

- The diaphragm is seen as a bright white curved structure (specular pattern of reflection) above the liver and provides a good landmark.
- It is important to image the kidney in its longitudinal axis. If this view is not adequately obtained then the probe can be moved further back towards the mid-axillary line.

  Ultrasound is performed in real time and minute adjustments of the transducer can be made in the orientation of the probe to obtain the best view of the hepatorenal space as a purely coronal view may provide a limited view.

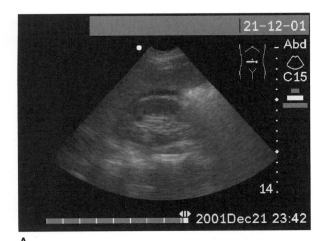

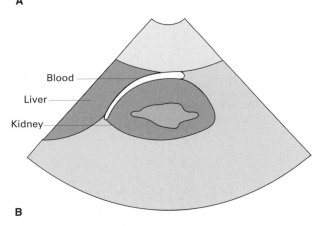

Figure 4.6 Perihepatic view. (**A**) Positive image. (**B**) Drawing.

- The ribs cast acoustic shadows, which may obscure the underlying anatomy. The probe may have to be moved and orientated to find an acoustic window between them.
- Beware of mistaking the inferior vena cava or gallbladder for free fluid.

Perisplenic view

The perisplenic window can be quite difficult to obtain as the spleen lies more superior and posterior than may be expected.

Patient Again a cooperative patient may be able to improve the view by taking a deep breath. Alternatively turning the patient slightly on to their right side, if injuries allow, may be useful.

Probe position

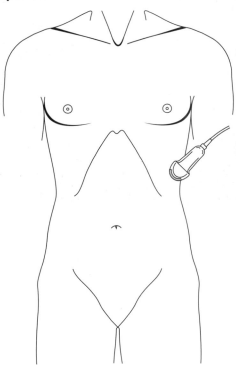

Figure 4.7 Perisplenic probe position. The probe must be placed along the posterior axillary line on the left side, in the most inferior two or three intercostal spaces. The best view is usually obtained with the transducer one or two spaces cephalad compared to the right side.

Points and pitfalls

- The left kidney can be used as a landmark as it will frequently be the first recognisable structure. In this situation the probe must be moved cephalad to visualise the spleen and gain a view of the interface between the two organs.
- The stomach and splenic flexure of the colon are anterior to the splenorenal space and may prevent good images being obtained if they contain air. A posterior position of the probe should avoid this.
- The transducer is angled obliquely and the spleen and kidney should be visible and fluid detected in the space between the two organs.
- The posterior subphrenic space is more dependent than the splenorenal fossa, therefore fluid will also collect in this recess between the spleen and diaphragm. The probe should be moved or angled further cephalad to obtain the desired image. Left sided pleural fluid can also be appreciated in this view.

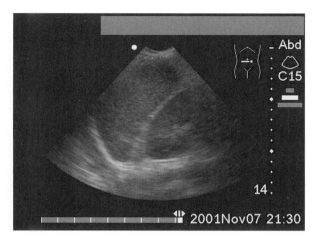

A

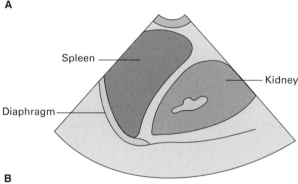

B

Figure 4.8 Perisplenic view. (**A**) Normal image.
(**B**) Drawing.

- Rib shadows can be difficult and may make it necessary to find an acoustic window between them.

Pelvis

Patient
Patient supine.

Points and pitfalls

- It is ideal to perform FAST before a catheter is inserted as a full bladder provides an ideal acoustic window for ultrasound.

  The bladder can be easily identified if it is full. However if the patient has voided or a catheter has been placed, the bladder is not seen.
- If a catheter is already *in situ*, sterile saline can be instilled into the bladder and the catheter clamped to allow visualisation.
- Alternatively the Foley balloon may be visible and can be used as a landmark.

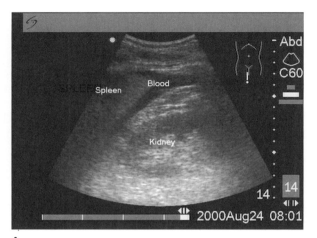

A

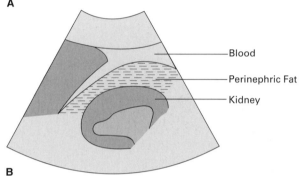

B

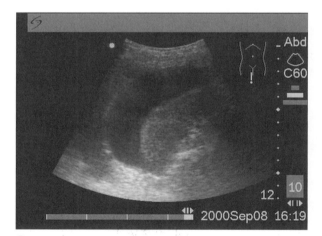

C

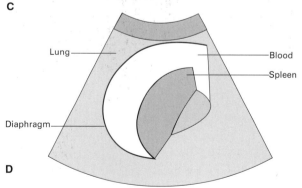

D

Figure 4.9 Perisplenic views. (**A**) and (**C**) Positive image.
(**B**) and (**D**) Drawings.

Probe position

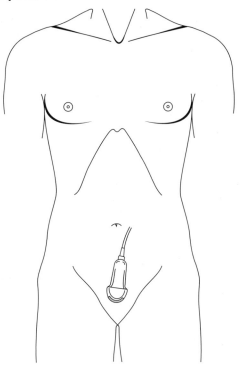

Figure 4.10   Pelvic probe position. The transducer is placed immediately above the symphysis pubis, initially longitudinally and then rotated transversely. The probe is then angled down into the pelvis to locate the bladder.

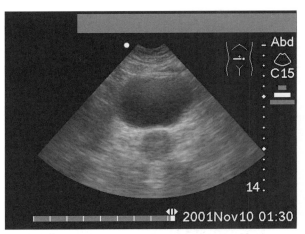

A

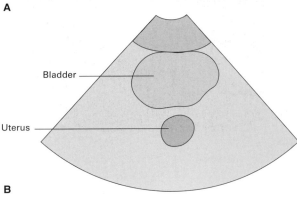

B

Figure 4.11   Pelvic view. (**A**) Normal image. (**B**) Drawing.

- When the bladder is identified the transducer is rotated to provide a transverse picture of the bladder.
- Fluid will be detected posterior to the bladder (Figure 4.12).
- If there is significant bleeding the bowel may be seen floating in the blood.
- Fluid within the bowel can be mistaken for free fluid. Peristaltic waves will cause a rhythmic movement of intraluminal fluid, which can help to differentiate it from free fluid.

Limitations

It is vital that those using FAST to assess the critically injured patient be aware of the limitations of the technology and technique. FAST augments but does not replace the clinical evaluation of the patient and the results must always be reviewed in the light of the clinical findings. FAST can produce suboptimal images for a number of reasons. Operator error is one of the leading causes. However obese body habitus, excessive bowel distension, subcutaneous emphysema, and poor contact between skin and transducer all reduce the quality of the images. Rib shadows and scanning artefacts will also reduce the diagnostic accuracy. *Any FAST scan that does not visualise all four regions is suboptimal and therefore inadequate.* An additional diagnostic test is required to exclude intra-abdominal bleeding in this situation.

Technical limitations
• Obesity
• Intestinal gas
• Subcutaneous emphysema

As with any diagnostic modality, clinical judgement must prevail, regardless of ultrasound results. This is particularly important in the initial phase of learning FAST, which must be undertaken as proctored examinations with appropriate mentoring.

Scoring systems

Attempts have been made to use scoring systems to quantify the amount of free intraperitoneal blood detected on FAST. These could potentially be used to support the decision to operate or undertake a non-operative policy. Neither system developed by Huang or McKenny has been shown to be reliable and further work is required if scoring systems to accurately quantify fluid and predict laparotomy are to be successfully incorporated into FAST protocols.

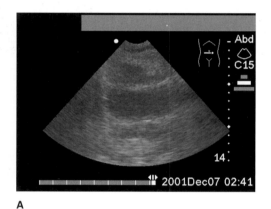

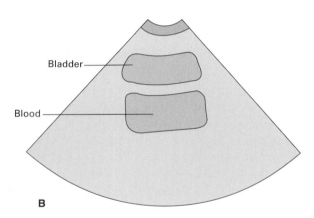

Figure 4.12 Pelvic view. (**A**) Positive image. (**B**) Drawing.

Disadvantages of FAST

FAST is limited by technical factors that affect image acquisition, operator errors, and errors in the interpretation of the images within the clinical scenario. The technical factors have been discussed above and may obscure one or all of the ultrasound windows. However even with satisfactory images, errors can arise as significant injuries may occur in the retroperitoneum (less well visualised) or with limited or no haemoperitoneum.

The negative FAST examination has been the subject of much debate and the topic was reviewed at the International Consensus Meeting. In isolation a negative FAST has limited value; it must be considered in conjunction with the clinical assessment and augmented either with a CT scan or a period of observation and a repeat FAST. This approach is included as a component of many trauma algorithms.

FAST algorithm

The immediate assessment of the trauma patient for haemorrhage occurs during the circulation phase of the primary survey. FAST scanning is a unique modality for the rapid evaluation of the trauma patient in the emergency room during this phase and should not interfere with the resuscitation process. Several algorithms based on FAST have been suggested based on the clinical stability of the patient. Our current algorithm for the evaluation of the patient with suspected blunt abdominal trauma is outlined. As discussed previously in this chapter FAST can be used for the assessment of all injured patients, and it is our practice to scan penetrating trauma as well as blunt trauma patients on arrival in ER as an initial triage.

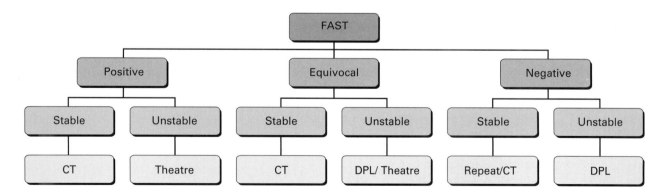

Figure 4.13   Blunt abdominal trauma algorithm.

Summary

FAST is gradually becoming accepted as the initial investigation of choice in the trauma patient. In multiply injured unstable patients FAST provides a rapid triage of the abdomen and chest and can provide the emergency team with valuable information within seconds. The limitations of the technique must be recognised and results must always be interpreted within the context of the clinical findings. FAST is a "rule in" investigation; its value to "rule out" is far less assured.

Further reading

Dolich MO, McKenney MG, Varela JE, Compton RP, McKenney KL, Cohn S. 2576 ultrasounds for blunt abdominal trauma. *J Trauma*, 2001;**50**:108–12.

Rozycki GS, Oschner MG, Jaffin JH, Champion HR. Prospective evaluation of surgeons' use of ultrasound in the evaluation of trauma patients. *J Trauma* 1993; **34**:516–26.

Rozycki GS, Oschner MG, Schmidt JA, *et al.* A prospective study of surgeon-performed ultrasound as the primary adjuvant modality for injured patient assessment. *J Trauma* 1995;**39**:492–500.

Rozycki GS, Shackford S. Trauma Ultrasound for Surgeons. In Staren ED (ed) *Ultrasound for the Surgeon.* New York: Lipincott-Raven, 1997:120–35.

5 Ultrasound of the chest

*DOUGLAS R HAMILTON, ASHOT SARGYSAN,
SCOTT A DULCHAVSKY*

Objectives
- To introduce thoracic ultrasound
- To present the technique for ultrasound detection of pneumothorax and haemothorax
- To introduce further applications of thoracic ultrasound

Introduction

Pneumothorax is commonly associated with blunt or penetrating chest trauma or can spontaneously occur in susceptible patients. The incidence of pneumothorax is particularly high in patients in the intensive care unit, especially if they are on mechanical ventilation. The diagnosis of pneumothorax is suggested by clinical signs and symptoms and is generally confirmed by chest radiography. Haemothorax or hydrothorax can occur in patients with chest injury or secondary to a variety of medical conditions. The diagnosis of blood or fluid in the chest is generally apparent based on decreased breath sounds and dullness in the chest to percussion; the diagnosis is confirmed with radiography. Although the ability to obtain a chest radiograph is usually present without significant delay in the emergency room or hospital ward, occasionally, patient instability or difficulties in transport or radiographic availability require the diagnosis to be made clinically and definitive treatment accomplished before radiologic verification of these conditions.

Pneumothorax or haemothorax can also occur in patients in remote areas where radiographic evaluation is delayed or impossible, such as in military conflicts, rural medicine, or potentially during space exploration. Power, weight, and space requirements make radiography impractical in these applications; therefore, sound clinical diagnosis is paramount. Unfortunately, environmental effects such as noise and possibly limited training of health care providers in these situations further complicate the diagnosis of chest conditions.

Ultrasound has proven diagnostic accuracy in abdominal applications; however, it has not been widely used in the chest. Direct

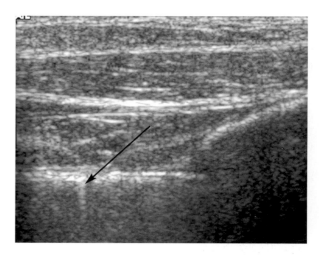

Figure 5.1 The comet tail artefact is seen as a hyper-echoid shadow which begins at the interpleural line and extends deep into the scanning window.

ultrasonographic evaluation of the lung is hampered by the high acoustic impedance of air-containing structures. Nonetheless, pneumothorax may be excluded on the basis of the somewhat paradoxical visualisation of artefacts resulting from the lung-chest wall interface. In a normal patient, a lung-chest wall interface or pleural line is seen that is accompanied by a to-and-fro sliding motion, "lung sliding" or "gliding", synchronised with respiration. A secondary finding, the comet tail artefact, is produced by highly reflective objects in the scanning field, such as water-rich structures in the lung, and manifests as an echogenic band that extends from the object deep into the field (Figure 5.1). The comet tail artefact is produced by the visceral pleura; therefore, the presence of this sign excludes pneumothorax. Although the comet tail artefact has been described in many patient populations, it is generally produced by small air collections or consolidation of the lung; therefore, the prevalence and utility of this finding in trauma patients is questionable. Furthermore, subcutaneous shotgun pellets or subcutaneous emphysema may cause the comet tail sign; therefore, caution must be exercised when interpreting this finding in trauma patients.

The ultrasound diagnosis of haemothorax is more conventional. Fluid in the pleural cavity is readily visualised as an echogenic, crescent shaped area in the most dependent area in the patient. Haemothorax is often seen during FAST (Focussed assessment with sonography for trauma) examinations when visualising the splenic and liver windows. The finding of supra-diaphragmatic fluid on this examination appears to be a sensitive and reliable indication that fluid or blood is present in the chest.

The first reported use of ultrasound to diagnose pneumothorax was in a veterinary journal, where pneumothorax in a horse was diagnosed, allowing percutaneous aspiration. Subsequently, over 100 cases of pneumothorax have been diagnosed by thoracic ultrasound, predominantly in isolated series. The technique has been examined in ventilated patients and after lung biopsy in Europe; however, it has not been widely evaluated in the United States.

Thoracic ultrasound for the detection of pneumothorax or haemothorax is a clinically attractive modality that can be readily learned with minimal instruction. The surface of the lung is easily visualised with a high-frequency probe and can be rapidly verified in the normal contra lateral chest. The scan can be concomitantly accomplished as other therapeutic manoeuvres are performed and it has a sensitivity comparable to or greater than radiography. The rediscovery of this technique, mandated by requirements of the space programme, suggests that trauma ultrasonographic evaluation should be broadened to include the thorax. The verification of thoracic ultrasound, coupled with newer, portable ultrasound equipment, may allow expanded application of ultrasound in clinical situations where radiography is difficult or impossible.

Ultrasound training and technique

Ultrasonographic evaluation of the chest can be accomplished with any standard ultrasound machine that is available in the emergency room or radiographic suite. Although adequate visualisation of the pleura can be accomplished with a mid-frequency range curvilinear probe, a linear transducer with a high frequency range (> 7 MHz) provides the greatest diagnostic accuracy. Ultrasound to exclude haemothorax is

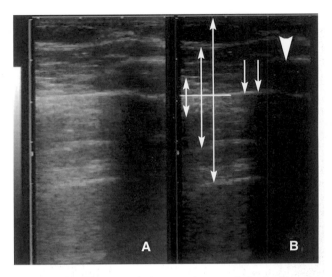

Figure 5.2 The normal ultrasound anatomic landmarks of the chest are readily visualised seen on this static image. The chest wall musculature, fascia, and the visceral-parietal interface should be easily discernable with a high frequency probe.

an extension of the classic abdominal FAST examination. The diaphragm can be visualised with a standard, curvilinear probe placed in the lateral abdominal positions to exclude fluid in Morison's Pouch or the splenorenal fossa. A haemothorax is seen as fluid in the supra-diaphragmatic space. Confirmation can be obtained by asking the patient to take a deep breath and visualising the fluid shift with diaphragmatic excursions.

Performance of a chest ultrasound examination for pneumothorax begins in the unaffected chest to gain familiarity with topography as well as establish a normal baseline. The linear probe is placed longitudinally over the anterior chest in the third or fourth intercostal space. The focal zone of the probe is maximised to visualise the pleural interface zone (generally 3–5 cm) (Figure 5.2). The intercostal plane is located by identifying the acoustic shadow of the rib in real time while the probe is displaced longitudinally (Figure 5.3). This discontinuous relief represents a constant landmark that facilitates visualisation of the pleura as a hyperechoic line between and below the ribs. Performance of the examination in the uninjured chest is especially important in novice ultrasonographers to determine a baseline and to affirm the normal ultrasound findings in patients without pneumothorax. The lung pleura is visualised between rib echogenic windows and observed for evidence of the to-and-fro "sliding"

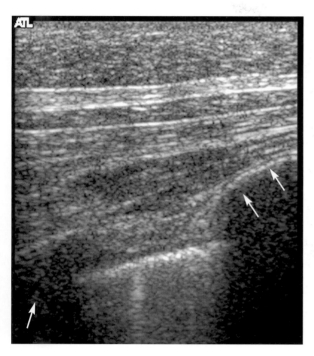

Figure 5.3 The rib is a stable orientation landmark which allows the visceral and parietal pleural interface to be identified. The ultrasound field can be optimised to this depth to allow maximum sensitivity of the examination.

sign on respiration and/or the "comet tail" artefact. The scan is then repeated in the contra lateral chest. The absence of "lung sliding" after an adequate window (30–60 seconds) infers a collapsed lung.

The technique is quickly learned by operators familiar with ultrasound use in abdominal trauma and adds less than two to three minutes to the total evaluation. Since the diagnosis of pneumothorax relies on the absence of normally present findings, operator recognition of lung sliding is essential, suggesting that scanning of the thoracic cavity should be incorporated into routine abdominal evaluations to increase familiarity.

There are key technical points of thoracic ultrasound that deserve mention. First, there is consensus that high-frequency transducers are required for optimal images and that dynamic images are required to differentiate pneumothorax from normal lung fields. Scanning should begin in the unaffected lung to confirm the presence of lung sliding. Probe placement is facilitated by identification of the echogenic rib in the lateral clavicular line in the third to fourth interspace and directing the probe inferiorly to

allow visualisation of lung sliding in the midportion of the viewing screen. After confirmation of lung sliding, the contra lateral chest is then scanned for the presence or absence of lung sliding for a number of respiratory cycles; cooperative patients are asked to increase their respiratory efforts.

Sensitivity and specificity of thoracic ultrasound

Moderate haemothorax is readily seen during the FAST examination. The detection threshold is not clear, however, animal experiments suggest that 150 cc of fluid can be reliably visualised with standard curvilinear probes.

The sensitivity of lung ultrasound in the detection of pneumothorax appears comparable to or perhaps greater than routine radiography. Prior investigators have attempted to correlate ultrasound findings with the size of the pneumothorax and found minimal correlation. Nonetheless, sensitivities greater than 90% have been reported in patients with pneumothorax. Unconfirmed data analysis from this trial and animal work suggest that modest pneumothorax can be diagnosed with visualisation of segmental lung sliding or localised areas of pleural nonvisualisation.

Thoracic ultrasound has been shown to accurately diagnose pneumothorax in a variety of applications. However, the accuracy of thoracic ultrasound, performed by non-radiologists, to exclude pneumothorax was not known. Therefore, to define the utility of ultrasound of the chest performed by surgeons, we performed a retrospective evaluation of thoracic ultrasound at Detroit Receiving Hospital. Patients were actively enrolled in the study over the period 1 July 1999 to 1 March 2000. There were 382 patients who fulfilled inclusion criteria during the enrolment period and had ultrasound of the thorax performed. The majority were male patients (74%), and the injury demographics of the patient population reflected an urban Level I trauma centre.

Pleural lung sliding was readily visualised in all of the patients without a pneumothorax (343 of 382), for a true-negative rate of 100%. There were no comet tail artefacts noted in this patient subgroup. The ultrasonic examination was suboptimal in one patient with a spontaneous pneumothorax and one patient with blunt chest trauma and rib fractures. Both of these patients had moderate subcutaneous emphysema, which made the examination considerably more difficult. If these patients are included in the analysis, the sensitivity or true-positive rate is 95% (p = 0·0001 by analysis of variance [ANOVA]). One patient had an initial negative chest radiograph and a positive ultrasound examination after a stab wound to the chest; a repeat chest radiograph four hours later demonstrated an apical pneumothorax. Although this patient may not have had a pneumothorax on initial ultrasound evaluation, an alternative explanation is that the ultrasound correctly identified a small pneumothorax below the detection threshold of portable radiography. This finding has been corroborated by other investigators and correlated with CT of the chest.

Rib fractures were occasionally demonstrated in some of the patients during the thoracic ultrasound examination. Modest pressure on the transducer overlying the contused or fractured rib was well tolerated by the patients; a presumptive diagnosis of rib fracture was inferred when cortical discontinuity or a constant transverse echogenic line was noted in the rib. Lung sliding may be absent in patients without pneumothorax who have extensive pleural scarring or adult respiratory distress syndrome; the ultrasonic diagnosis of pneumothorax in these patients appears to be considerably more challenging.

Not all reports have been without caution. Sistrom reported a high interobserver variability and a positive predictive value of only 40% in diagnosing pneumothorax on the basis of a retrospective videotape review.[25] Lin *et al* attempted to correlate ultrasound findings with the size of the pneumothorax and found minimal correlation. Unfortunately, this study used archived tapes of the examination, which did not allow the operator to compare the two hemithoraces or to investigate subtle findings in the chest, suggesting that a trained operator in attendance is essential. Nonetheless, sensitivities greater than 90% have been reported in patients with pneumothorax. These findings seem to emphasise that both ultrasonographic examination and normal lung excursion are dynamic processes that require real-time imaging (because of the high degree of operator dependence) and real-time interpretation (to observe lung sliding and comet tail artefact).

Colour power Doppler thoracic ultrasound

Conventional duplex Doppler ultrasound depicts both direction and velocity of flow. Power colour Doppler (also known as amplitude-encoded colour Doppler) analyses and integrates movement regardless of flow velocity or direction and is superior for identifying low-velocity or low-volume flow (or motion). The ultrasound criteria currently used to exclude pneumothorax require dynamic, real-time imaging, which makes teletransmission or post-examination review difficult. Power colour Doppler may allow dynamic "lung sliding" to be effectively communicated with a single still image which would reduce requirements for image storage, documentation, transmission, and interpretation.

The absence of a power colour Doppler signal (the "power slide") at the thoracopleural interface may serve as an additional criterion to identify pneumothorax. The technique requires an ultrasound device capable of power colour Doppler imaging with a high frequency linear array transducer (7 to 10 MHz range). The linear probe is placed to visualise the thoracopleural interface as in routine thoracic ultrasound. The colour power Doppler signal is then activated and the power gain is gradually increased. In a normal lung there will be a flow signal beginning at the interpleural interface corresponding to the gliding or sliding movement of the two pleural surfaces excluding pneumothorax. There will be no colour power Doppler signal seen in patients with a pneumothorax, rather, as the signal gain is increased, spurious noise will be seen in all layers of the image. The transducer must be held in a fixed location during the examination to avoid motion artefacts, which can be erroneously interpreted as pleural sliding.

Thoracic ultrasound: future applications

Increased user familiarity and skill has allowed ultrasound to be incorporated into routine emergency patient care by non-radiologist physicians in select applications. Recent studies further suggest that the use of ultrasound may be expanded to include additional indications (extremity trauma, sinusitis, ocular trauma, vascular injury, dental infections, etc) where

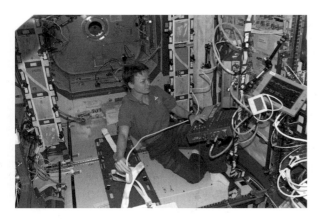

Figure 5.4 The NASA Human Research Facility Ultrasound Unit is shown onboard the International Space Station. The machine is a flight modified ATL 5000 ultrasound system and is equipped with a variety of probes.

radiologic assessments are delayed or impractical. Ongoing clinical trials will provide verifiable data to determine the accuracy of these techniques to allow future incorporation into clinical practice where appropriate. Military or aerospace paradigms have novel constraints and provide test beds to assess this technology for later incorporation into general clinical practice.

Medical care capabilities for the International Space Station (ISS) and future exploratory class space missions are currently being defined. Numerous human health risks have been identified which include microgravity-specific health concerns as well as routine medical care. Although rigorous astronaut selection procedures reduce the chance of chronic health problems, acute conditions can occur especially during extended duration space flight. The ISS Medical Operations Requirements Document requires that "the capability to diagnose and treat anticipated routine medical and dental problems shall be provided."

The NASA Critical Path Roadmap Project coordinated a consensus conference of health care experts who rated trauma as the highest impact on incidence versus mission and health. The feasibility of ultrasonic imaging in human space flight has been demonstrated in preliminary investigations on both American and Russian spacecraft. NASA-Medical Operations have demonstrated the utility of diagnostic abdominal, retroperitoneal, and thoracic ultrasound in micro gravity experiments on animal models during parabolic flight on KC-135 aircraft. These

investigations suggest the sensitivity and specificity of ultrasound in this application are not degraded during microgravity conditions and may be enhanced in certain circumstances.

The medical equipment onboard the ISS is manifested as part of the American Crew Health Care System or the Russian medical hardware system. However, certain additional medical hardware is also available on ISS as part of the ISS Human Research Facility (HRF) (Figure 5.4). The specific hardware requirements to expand the operational use of ultrasound in space are being defined. The HRF Ultrasound System is an advanced, multipurpose, diagnostic imaging tool and is equipped with a reasonable array of ultrasound probes which could significantly enhance the ability to timely diagnose, stage, and monitor a wide variety of serious conditions. The outcome of a medical contingency may be changed drastically, and an unnecessary evacuation may be prevented, if clinical decisions are supported by objective diagnostic information. The HRF Ultrasound system is the only diagnostic imaging device currently manifested on ISS; the use of ultrasound in epidemiologically defined clinical conditions may provide additional information in many clinical situations to support the Crew Health Care System/the Integrated Medical System of the Station.

We recently completed a proctored complete ultrasound examination of an Expedition 5 crew member on the International Space Station (Sargysan AE *et al*, in preparation). Crew member Peggy Whitson performed an ultrasound self-examination which included a FAST and thoracic ultrasound exam with audio direction from experts in Mission Control (Figure 5.5). On site and down linked image quality was excellent and would have provided essential information to guide clinical decision making. This initial ultrasound experience suggests that limited crew member training, combined with directed guidance from ground based experts using visual and audio cues, provides an effective paradigm to complete a complicated medical task. The examination was conducted using limited bandwidth constraints which would facilitate reproduction in terrestrial situations such as rural medicine. It is anticipated that two way video proctoring, although not essential, would augment more complex procedures or examinations.

Although some of the aerospace medical procedures currently investigated by NASA are appropriate only for the space environment, many

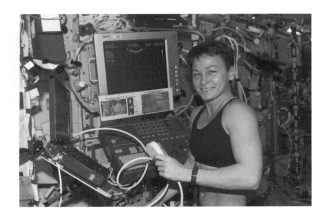

Figure 5.5 Expedition 5 crew-member Peggy Whitson is shown completing an ultrasound self examination in the HRF on the International Space Station. The images and video were down-linked realtime to Mission Control in Houston, Texas for evaluation.

of the diagnostic and therapeutic algorithms are readily transferable to terrestrial medicine including rural or military applications. The expanded use of diagnostic ultrasound is advantageous as it is readily available (hand-held portable devices), requires only modest training for image acquisition/interpretation, and does not expose the patient to ionising radiation.[9] The widespread verification of remotely guided ultrasound examinations, performed by first responders or similarly trained personnel, would provide a significant, clinically relevant advance in space medical capabilities with profound Earth-based ramifications in rural and military applications.

Summary

Ultrasound of the chest is quickly learnt by operators familiar with ultrasound use in abdominal trauma and adds less than two to three minutes to the total evaluation. Since the diagnosis of pneumothorax relies on the absence of normally present findings, operator recognition of lung sliding is essential, suggesting that scanning of the thoracic cavity should be incorporated into routine abdominal evaluations to increase familiarity. Key technical points include the use of high-frequency transducers to obtain optimal images and that dynamic images are required to differentiate pneumothorax from normal lung fields. Scanning should begin in the normal lung to confirm the presence of lung sliding. Probe placement is facilitated by identification of the echogenic rib in

the lateral axillary line in the third to fourth interspace and directing the probe inferiorly to allow visualisation of lung sliding. Colour power Doppler visualisation of "power sliding" may facilitate the diagnosis and simplify documentation of the finding. The rediscovery of thoracic ultrasound, mandated by requirements of the space programme, suggests that trauma ultrasonographic evaluation should be broadened to include the thorax. The verification of thoracic ultrasound, coupled with newer, portable ultrasound equipment, may allow expanded application of ultrasound in clinical situations where radiography is difficult or impossible.

Further reading

Chiles C, Ravin CE. Radiographic recognition of pneumothorax in the intensive care unit. *Crit Care Med* 1986;**14(8)**:677–80.

Cunningham J, Kirkpatrick AW, Nicolaou S, *et al.* Enhanced Recognition of "Lung Sliding" with Power Colour Doppler Imaging in the Diagnosis of Pneumothorax. *J Trauma* 2002;**52**:769–71.

Dulchavsky SA, Hamilton DR, Diebel LN, Sargsyan AE, Billica RD, Williams DR. Thoracic Ultrasound Diagnosis of Pneumothorax. *J Trauma* 1999;**47**:970.

Dulchavsky SA, Schwarz KL, Kirkpatrick AW, *et al.* Prospective Evaluation of Thoracic Ultrasound in the Detection of Pneumothorax. *J Trauma* 2001;**50**:201–5.

Goodman TR, Traill ZC, Phillips AJ, Berger J, Gleeson FV. Ultrasound detection of pneumothorax. *Clin Radiol* 1999;**B**:736–9.

Kirkpatrick AW, Brown DR, Crickmer S, *et al.* Hand-held portable sonography for the on-mountain exclusion of a pneumothorax. *Wilderness Environ Med* 2000;**12(4)**:270–2.

Kirkpatrick AW, Ng AK, Dulchavsky SA, *et al.* Sonographic diagnosis of a pneumothorax inapparent on plain radiography: confirmation by computed sonography. *J Trauma* 2001;**50(4)**:750–2.

Kirkpatrick AW, Simons RK, Brown R, Nicolaou S, Dulchavsky SA. The hand-held FAST: experience with hand-held trauma sonography in a level-I urban trauma center. *Injury* 2002;**33(4)**:303–8.

Krejci CS, Trent EJ, Dubinsky T. Thoracic sonography. *Respir Care* 2001;**46(9)**:932–9.

Lichtenstein DA, Menu Y. A bedside ultrasound sign ruling out pneumothorax in the critically ill. *Chest* 1995;**108**:1345–8.

Lichtenstein DA, Meziere G, Biderman P, Gepner A. The comet tail artefact: an ultrasound sign ruling out pneumothorax. *Intensive Care Med* 1999;**25**:383–8.

Lichtenstein D, Meziere G. Ultrasound probably has a bright future in the diagnosis of pneumothorax. *J Trauma* 2002;**52(3)**:607.

Lin MS, Hwang JJ, *et al.* Ultrasonography of chest diseases: analysis of 154 cases. *Gaoxiong Yi Xue Ke Xue Za Zhi* 1992;**8(10)**:525–34.

Ma OJ, Mateer JR. Trauma ultrasound examination versus chest radiography in the detection of haemothorax. *Ann Emerg Med* 1997;**29(3)**:312–5; discussion 315–6.

Melton S, Beck G, Hamilton D, *et al.* How to test a medical technology for space: trauma sonography in microgravity. McGill Med J (In press).

Polk JD, Fallon WF Jr, Kovach B, *et al.* The "Airmedical F.A.S.T." for trauma patients – the initial report of a novel application for sonography. *Aviat Space Environ Med* 2001;**72(5)**:432–6.

Ratanen NW. Diagnostic ultrasound: diseases of the thorax. *Vet Clin North Am* 1986;**2**:49–66.

Rozycki GS, Feliciano DV, Davis TP. Ultrasound as used in thoracoabdominal trauma. *Surg Clin North Am* 1998;**78(2)**:295–310.

Rozycki GS, Ochsner MG, *et al.* Early detection of hemoperitoneum by ultrasound examination of the right upper quadrant: a multicenter study. *J Trauma* 1998;**45(5)**:878–83.

Sargsyan AE, Hamilton DR, Nicolaou S, *et al.* Ultrasound evaluation of the magnitude of pneumothorax: a new concept. *Am Surg* 2001;**67(3)**:232–6.

Sisley AC, Rozycki GS, Ballard RB, *et al.* Rapid detection of traumatic effusion using surgeon-performed ultrasonography. *J Trauma* 1998;**44(2)**:291–6; discussion 296–7.

Sistrom CL, Reiheld CT, Spencer BG, Wallace KK. Detection and estimation of the volume of pneumothorax using real-time ultrasonography. *Am J Roentgenol* 1996;**166**:317–21.

Targhetta R, Bourgeois JM, Chavagneux R, *et al.* Ultrasonographic approach to diagnosing hydro-pneumothorax. *Chest* 1992;**101(4)**:931–4.

Targhetta R, Bourgeois JM, Balmes P. Echography of pneumothorax. *Rev Mal Respir* 1990;**7**:575–9.

Targhetta R, Bourgeois JM, Chavagneux R, Balmes P. Diagnosis of pneumothorax by ultrasound immediately after ultrasonically guided aspiration biopsy. *Chest* 1992;**101**:855–6.

Wernecke K, Galanski M, Peters PE, Hansen J. [Sonographic diagnosis of pneumothorax.] *ROFO Fortschr Geb Rontgenstr Nuklearmed* 1989;**150(1)**:84–5.

Wernecke K, Galanski M, Peters PE, Hansen J. Pneumothorax: evaluation by ultrasound – preliminary results. *J Thorac Imaging* 1987;**7**:76–78.

Ziskin MC, Thickman DI, Goldenberg NJ, *et al.* The comet tail artefact. *J Ultrasound Med* 1982;**1(1)**:1–7.

6 Ultrasound assessment of the abdominal aorta

SIMON ENGLAND

Objectives
- To revise abdominal aortic anatomy
- To define the technique of scanning the abdominal aorta
- To introduce the ultrasound findings of aortic aneurysms

Introduction

Rupture of an abdominal aortic aneurysm is a relatively common vascular surgical emergency, with rupture rates in the over 50s of 76 per 100 000 patient years for men and 11 per 100 000 in women. The incidence of abdominal aneurysm is reported to be up to 117 per 100 000 with the peak incidence seen in males in the ninth decade. The majority of acute ruptures are clinically obvious with severe back and abdominal pain, shock, and an expansile abdominal mass being the most frequent clinical manifestations. Most vascular surgeons will subject the patient to operative repair, without imaging data, on clinical grounds alone. Infrequently the clinical presentation is less obvious and a contained or subacute leak is suspected. In these circumstances, ultrasound can identify the aneurysm but often does not demonstrate a peri-aortic haematoma. CT is a better modality to identify these cases. The strength of ultrasound lies in its ability to diagnose an abdominal aortic aneurysm using a quick, easy, non-invasive, accurate and bedside technique. Ultrasound is thus of great utility in the assessment of the abdominal aorta in patients with non-traumatic haemorrhagic shock in the absence of obvious clinical signs in the abdomen. This strategy clearly expedites the diagnosis, leading to emergent surgery offering the best chance of survival.

Abdominal aortic anatomy

The aorta enters the abdomen in the midline under the median arcuate ligament at the level of T12. It proceeds inferiorly in the retroperitoneum on the anterior aspects of the lumbar vertebral bodies to its bifurcation point at the level of L4 just to the left of midline. The major branches are the coeliac axis, T12, the superior mesenteric artery, L1, and the renal arteries, L1. Its right side is closely related to the IVC. Anteriorly it is related from above, downwards to the liver, the left renal vein, the pancreatic body, the duodenal third part, the root of the small bowel mesentery, and small bowel loops.

With increasing age the aorta frequently dilates, elongates (ectasia), and becomes tortuous but the infrarenal diameter should not exceed 3 cm.

Surface anatomy

Midline epigastrium to $\simeq$ 1 cm below and left of umbilicus.

Scan technique/equipment

Choose a probe suitable for general abdominal imaging, usually a sector or curvilinear 3 to 5 MHz transducer optimised to aortic depth. Expose the abdomen, whilst maintaining the patient's dignity. Place the probe in the upper midline and obtain a longitudinal section of the aorta. The imaging convention is that cranial structures are presented on the left side of the screen. It may

Retroperitoneal vascular anatomy	
• **AA**	Abdominal aorta
• **CA**	Coeliac axis
• **CHA**	Common hepatic artery
• **CIA**	Common iliac artery
• **CIV**	Common iliac vein
• **EIA**	External iliac artery
• **EIV**	External iliac vein
• **HV**	Hepatic vein
• **IVC**	Inferior vena cava
• **LRA and RRA**	Left and right renal arteries
• **LRV and RRV**	Left and right renal veins
• **SA**	Splenic artery
• **SMA**	Superior mesenteric artery

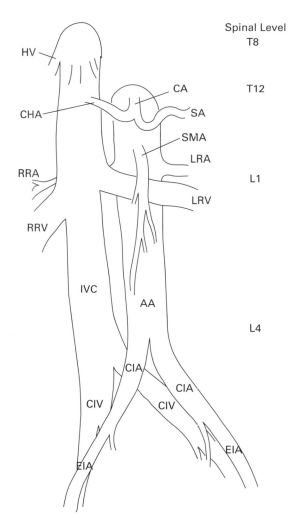

Spinal Level
T8

T12

L1

L4

Figure 6.1   Retroperitoneal vascular anatomy.
AA, abdominal aorta; IVC, inferior vena cava; CA, coeliac axis;
SA, splenic artery; CHA, common hepatic artery; SMA,
superior mesenteric artery; CIA, common iliac artery; EIA,
external iliac artery; LRA, left renal artery; RRA, right renal
artery; LRV, left renal vein; RRV, right renal vein; HV, hepatic
vein; CIV, common iliac vein; external iliac vein.

require some minor translational movements or
rotatory probe movements to optimise the
insonation plane into the plane of the aorta. The
aorta is recognised by its pulsation, definite
echogenic wall, branch pattern, and relationships
to adjacent structures.

By keeping the probe in the same plane the
probe is then moved caudally, erring slightly to
the left of midline to obtain a longitudinal section
of the lower aorta.

Measurement cursors are applied to the leading
and trailing aortic walls, perpendicular to the
long axis of the aorta to obtain measurement data.

The aorta may be tortuous, in which case
rotatory movements around the vertical axis

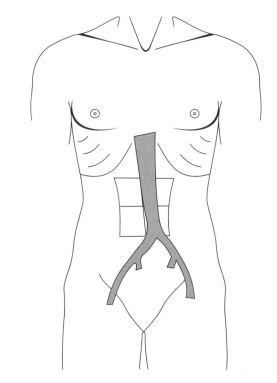

Figure 6.2   The surface anatomy of the abdominal aorta.

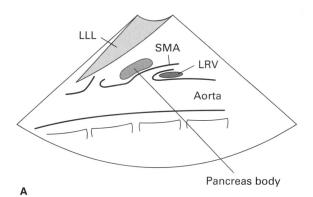

A

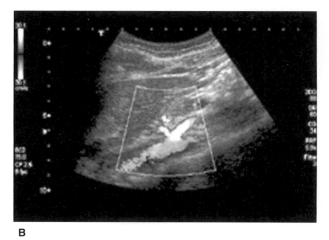

B

Figure 6.3   The normal aorta in longitudinal
section – upper abdomen. LLL, left lobe of liver.

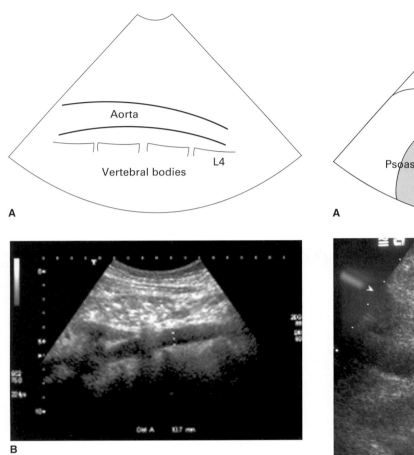

A

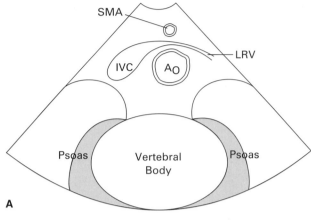

A

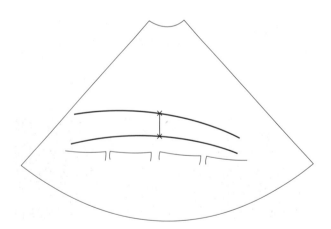

B

Figure 6.4 The normal aorta in longitudinal section – lower abdomen

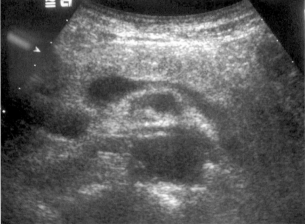

B

Figure 6.6 The normal upper abdominal aorta in transverse section

Figure 6.5 Correct application of measurement cursors.

of the probe will be necessary to optimise the longitudinal section. By rotating the probe slightly at the bifurcation, longitudinal views of the common iliac arteries are usually possible.

Next the aorta is imaged in the axial plane. The probe orientation is changed by rotating (anticlockwise) 90 degrees such that the imaging convention of the patient's right side to left side of screen is satisfied. In the upper midline, a representative section is shown in figure 6.6. By maintaining this probe orientation, translatory sweep movements along the midline will demonstrate the abdominal aorta in transverse section, from its origin to bifurcation, in a good subject. Again slight rotatory movements may be necessary to optimise orthogonal imaging if there is tortuosity. On completion wipe off the gel to minimise chilling the patient.

Normal findings

The aorta is usually well visualised as an anechoic pulsating structure, with easily resolvable walls, extending from the upper midline to the bifurcation. The major branches are usually easily identified, as are the proximal

Table 6.1 Location of aorta versus inferior vena cava

	Aorta	IVC
Extent	T12 → L4	T8 → L4/5
Position	Midline → left paramedian	Right paramedian
Walls	Distinct, echogenic, atheroma, thrombus	Barely resolvable
Pulsation	One visible per cycle	Two visible per cycle
Branch pattern	CA and SMA	HV
Relations	LEFT of CAVA	RIGHT of AORTA
Proximal connections	Lost above diaphragm	Heart (RA)
Doppler	Arterial waveform, flow distally	Venous waveform flow proximally

common iliacs. Mild tortuosity is common in the elderly and aortic atheroma is the norm, frequently calcified, which appears very echogenic and may "shadow". The infrarenal aorta (that is, below L1) measures less than 3 cm in diameter and there should not be a focal dilatation of the aorta > 50% of the diameter of the adjacent aorta.

Pitfalls

Make sure you are examining the aorta *NOT* the IVC (Table 6.1). Access difficulty, bowel gas, and obesity are the common problems. Increasing probe pressure, judicious angulation, acoustic window selection, and equipment optimisation can help but infrequently it is simply not possible to interrogate the relevant area.

Abdominal aortic aneurysms

The vast majority of abdominal aortic aneurysms are classified as degenerative or atherosclerotic. Mostly they are confined to the infrarenal abdominal aorta but can be found in conjunction with thoracic, iliac, femoral, and popliteal aneurysms. The risk of rupture is related to size with an exponential rise in the 5 to 6 cm diameter range.

Estimates of risk of rupture range from 5% per annum for a 5 cm aneurysm to 50% for a > 8 cm aneurysm. Hypertension, chronic obstructive pulmonary disease (COPD), and smoking are independent risk factors. Most ruptured

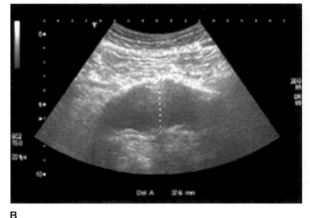

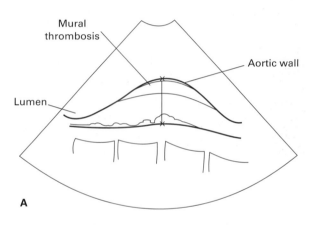

Figure 6.7 Abdominal aneurysm – longitudinal section

aneurysms are thus in the > 6 cm diameter range but, despite this, nearly 10% of ruptured aneurysms do not present with a palpable mass. This can be encountered in patients with extreme hypotension or in very obese patients.

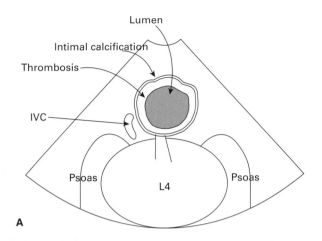

Lumen

Intimal calcification

Thrombosis

IVC

Psoas   L4   Psoas

A

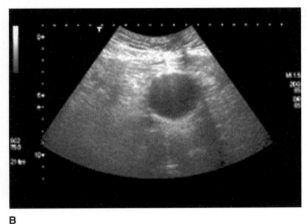

B

Figure 6.8   Abdominal aneurysm – transverse section.

Abdominal aneurysms can be sacular rather than fusiform, mycotic, dissecting, anastomotic pseudo aneurysm, and traumatic. Aneurysms in other vessels, for example internal and external iliac, splenic, renal, and other visceral arteries can also present with rupture. These entities are outside the scope of this chapter.

Ultrasound findings in abdominal aortic aneurysms

Using the techniques described above, the abdominal aorta is examined throughout its length in longitudinal and axial (transverse) planes. Aneurysms are almost always associated with tortuosity and it is usual that some complex probe angulations will be necessary to obtain an accurate measurement of maximum diameter.

The extent of the aneurysm is difficult to assess proximally as the renal artery origins are difficult to identify. Distal extent is usually easily defined and may extend beyond the bifurcation into the common iliac origins.

The important observations are the presence of pathological aortic dilatation and the maximum diameter. Measurement cursors should be placed on the leading and trailing aortic walls at the point of maximum dilatation perpendicular to the long axis of the aorta.

The aneurysm sac almost always contains thrombus, and intimal calcifications are commonly seen. The flowing lumen is anechoic, the thrombus variously echogenic, and the intimal calcifications strongly echogenic with acoustic shadowing. The appearances on the transverse images reflect this concentric layered structure.

The IVC may be compressed by the aneurysm sac and difficult to visualise.

Ultrasound can be of value in the diagnosis of a rupture but does not exclude a contained leak, or indeed, on some occasions, a large retroperitoneal collection. In view of this, CT is the preferred modality to make this diagnosis but if in the course of an ultrasound assessment an aneurysm is detected, intraperitoneal fluid or a retroperitoneal collection is strong circumstantial evidence of a rupture.

Summary

- The abdominal aorta is easily amenable to ultrasound interrogation in the majority of subjects.
- Abdominal aneurysms are relatively common and the rupture risk is related to size.
- Most ruptured aneurysms are clinically evident but 10% may not have a palpable, pulsatile mass.
- Most aneurysms are degenerative, infrarenal, abdominal, and fusiform.
- Abdominal aneurysms are easy to detect on abdominal ultrasound.
- Ultrasound is good at assessing the abdominal aorta in the emergency department.
- Aortic ultrasound is of value in assessing patients with occult hypovolaemia.
- Aneurysm extent, rupture, or contained leaks are best assessed with CT.

7 Abdominal emergencies

ALI NARAGHI, OTTO CHAN

Objectives
- To introduce ultrasound for abdominal emergencies
- To discuss the technique of ultrasound imaging for common acute abdominal problems

Introduction

Ultrasound in general has been relatively under-utilised in the immediate investigation and management of patients presenting to the accident and emergency department with abdominal symptoms. Whilst other modalities such as computed tomography may be more appropriate in some settings such as acute abdomen, ultrasound has several advantages which make it an invaluable tool in the work-up of those with abdominal complaints. It is a quick and cheap examination, which can be carried out at the bedside, thus allowing immediate assessment of patients without the need to move those who require monitoring. Its multiplanar and real time capabilities are ideally suited for evaluation of the abdominal organs and with its lack of ionising radiation, it is a suitable technique in all age groups and allows for repeat examinations to be performed. However, of all the imaging techniques, ultrasound is perhaps the most operator-dependent and therefore a thorough and systematic approach is required to ensure that subtle but significant abnormalities are not overlooked.

This chapter will describe the sonographic appearance of the common abdominal pathologies that may be encountered in the casualty department.

Pleural effusion

Although this is strictly not an abdominal condition, it often co-exists with other abdominal disorders such as subphrenic collections, acute pancreatitis, and peritonitis. Furthermore, basal pulmonary pathology may result in abdominal symptomatology.

The pleural space may be examined via an abdominal or an intercostal approach. Using

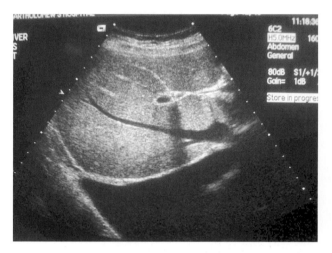

Figure 7.1 Pleural effusion: Anechoic fluid collection in the chest bounded by the hemidiaphragm inferiorly.

the abdominal approach the hemidiaphragms are visualised as echogenic curvilinear structures, superior to the liver and spleen. Pleural fluid is manifested as an anechoic or echo poor collection above the hemidiaphragms (Figure 7.1). Using the intercostal approach the anechoic collection is seen to lie between the echogenic air-filled lung, with its covering of visceral pleura, and the echogenic parietal pleura deep to the ribs. The ribs are identified as curvilinear echogenic structures casting an intense acoustic shadow. The underlying collapsed or consolidated lung may be seen as a triangular echogenic structure floating in the fluid.

Simple pleural effusions, in general, demonstrate no internal echoes. However, this does not exclude infection within the effusion. Complex collections such as haemothoraces and pleural empyemas may have internal echoes and septations. Septations are demonstrated as linear echogenic structures within the fluid. In such cases careful examination of the parietal pleura may demonstrate thickening.

Ascites

Accumulation of fluid in the peritoneal cavity may be seen in a wide variety of conditions. Ultrasound is exquisitely sensitive in detection of free intraperitoneal fluid. This fluid preferentially

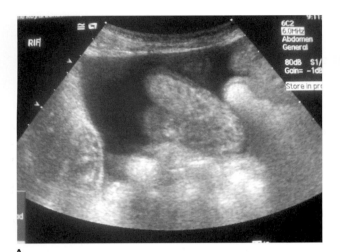

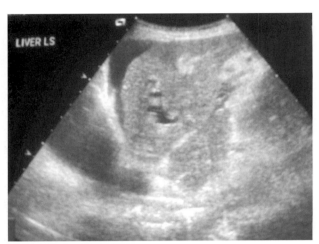

Figure 7.3 Subphrenic collection containing internal echoes lying in between the hemidiaphragm and liver.

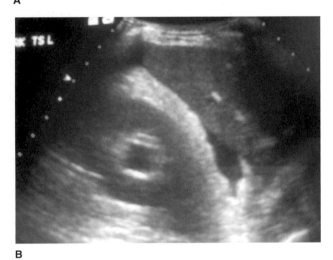

Figure 7.2 Free anechoic fluid within the peritoneal cavity consistent with ascites.

accumulates in the most dependent portions of the abdominal and pelvic cavity. These are the subphrenic spaces, particularly the right, the hepatorenal pouch of Morrison, the paracolic gutters, and the pelvic cul-de-sac with fluid being located posterior and superior to the bladder (Figure 7.2). With larger volumes of ascites, fluid may be seen in the small bowel mesentery with loops of small bowel floating within the ascites. Ascitic fluid may be anechoic or may possess internal echoes especially in the presence of blood and infection. Ultrasound can be used to guide aspiration and drainage.

Abdominal collections

Abdominal collections most commonly occur in the post-operative setting, following perforation of an abdominal viscus or secondary to trauma. They may contain blood or infected material. They are typically seen in the subphrenic spaces, the lesser sac, the paracolic gutters, and the pelvis.

Abdominal collections, particularly if complicated by haemorrhage or infection, contain internal echoes. Their shape and margins are partly dependent on adjacent structures. For example, subphrenic collections are typically crescentic in shape bounded by a linear echogenic hemidiaphragm superiorly and the liver or spleen inferiorly (Figure 7.3). Lower abdominal and pelvic collections may be indented by adjacent bowel. Distinction from bowel is made by the lack of peristalsis, the shape of the collection, and the nature of the wall. The wall of the collection may be variable in appearance ranging from a smooth thin wall to an irregular thick wall.

Liver ultrasound

Fatty liver

Increased accumulation of fat may be seen in the liver in a variety of conditions. These include obesity, diabetes mellitus, excess alcohol intake, and Cushing's syndrome. Normally the liver is slightly more echogenic than the adjacent renal parenchyma. With fatty infiltration there is progressive increased echogenicity of the liver parenchyma. This is demonstrated as an echogenic liver in comparison with the renal

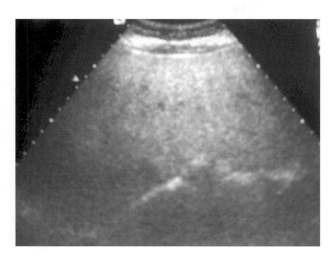

Figure 7.4 Diffusely increased liver echogenicity in fatty infiltration.

parenchyma. Secondary signs include impaired visualisation of the normally echogenic walls of the portal vein tributaries and difficulty in visualising the posterior aspects of the hepatic parenchyma which appear dark and with loss of anatomical detail. This is particularly so in more advanced cases and is due to increased attenuation of the ultrasound beam by the fatty liver (Figure 7.4).

Fatty involvement may be diffuse or patchy giving a geographical pattern or a more focal appearance in which case it may simulate a mass lesion. However, in focal fatty involvement, as opposed to a space occupying lesion, there is no alteration of liver contour and there is no mass effect with no displacement of hepatic vessels.

Infections

Acute hepatitis

Infectious hepatitis is a diagnosis that is confirmed by laboratory investigations. In most cases the sonographic appearances of the liver remain normal in acute hepatitis. Abnormal findings, which may be seen in hepatitis, include hepatomegaly, and generalised reduction in hepatic parenchymal echogenicity (the dark liver sign) associated with a cuff of increased echogenicity surrounding the portal triads. The portal triads normally demonstrate increased echogenicity, but this is accentuated and thickened in acute hepatitis. A secondary sign, which may also be present occasionally, is thickening of the gallbladder wall. However, the main role of ultrasound in acute hepatitis is to exclude other causes for derangement of liver function.

Hepatic abscess

Pyogenic abscesses may complicate other causes of intra-abdominal sepsis such as appendicitis, diverticulitis, or may result from biliary tract obstruction and sepsis. Classically pyogenic liver abscesses appear as cystic intrahepatic fluid collections with a thick wall. Commonly the collection is not completely anechoic but rather hypo-echoic with low level internal echoes. However, there can be a great variation in the appearance of pyogenic abscesses depending on the contents and degree of maturation. Sonographic appearances can vary from an anechoic collection to areas of slightly altered and usually hypo-echoic echotexture or to an echogenic lesion. The majority of lesions however demonstrate posterior acoustic enhancement. Similarly the wall thickness and regularity may vary.

Entamoeba histolytica classically infects the right colon and may spread to the liver via the portal venous system. Amoebic abscesses are classically seen in the right lobe of the liver. Although there are no specific sonographic features that allow differentiation between pyogenic and amoebic abscesses, the lack of wall echoes, uniform hypo-echoic reflectivity and subcapsular location are more frequent in amoebic abscesses. If there is a clinical suspicion of amoebic involvement, serological tests should be undertaken.

Hepatic involvement in hydatid disease caused by *Echinococcus granulosus* can also have a variable appearance. These include a simple completely cystic lesion, a cystic lesion with internal dependent echoes consistent with hydatid sand, a cystic lesion with linear echogenic strands representing separation of membranes, or multiple daughter cysts within a cyst. More longstanding lesions may demonstrate calcification, and this favours a diagnosis of hydatid cyst rather than a simple cyst.

Cirrhosis

Cirrhosis is essentially a pathological diagnosis but certain sonographic features are suggestive of the diagnosis. The normal liver has a smooth contour with a fine uniform echotexture. In cirrhosis, there is diffuse increased echogenicity of the liver, due to fatty infiltration, associated with coarsening of the liver echotexture. Early in the course of the disease process, the liver and in particular the caudate lobe, may be enlarged. However, with disease progression fibrosis becomes the predominant pathological process and often a small liver ensues. With development of regenerating and dysplastic nodules, nodular foci may be visualised throughout the liver, resulting in an irregular surface contour. This is best appreciated in the presence of ascites.

With development of portal hypertension ascites, splenic enlargement (> 12 cm) and portosystemic collaterals may be demonstrated. The latter may be seen in the splenic and renal hila and adjacent to the falciform ligament. Using Doppler ultrasound, the normal variation of portal vein velocity with respiration may be lost in portal hypertension and there may be reversal of the normal flow becoming hepatofugal (away from the liver). There may be associated enlargement of the splenic and portal veins.

Focal space occupying lesions

Focal, non-infective, hepatic space occupying lesions may be divided into primary and secondary neoplasms with the former being further subdivided into benign and malignant lesions.

The commonest benign lesions of the liver include simple cysts, haemangiomas, focal nodular hyperplasia (FNH), and adenomas. The first two are by far the commonest lesions. Simple cysts are characterised by an anechoic lesion with posterior acoustic accentuation and an imperceptible wall. Fine septations may occasionally be seen within the lesion. Haemangiomas demonstrate a well defined margin and homogeneous increased reflectivity. As the tumour enlarges it may develop a more heterogeneous echotexture and in some cases may produce posterior acoustic enhancement. Hepatic adenomas and FNH are difficult to distinguish, both being well demarcated with a homogeneous echotexture, which may be hypo- or hyperechoic in relation to the rest of the liver. Both may demonstrate a hypo-echoic central scar.

The commonest malignant primary liver neoplasm is a hepatocellular carcinoma (HCC), which is frequently seen in close association with cirrhosis. The underlying cirrhosis may give the hepatic parenchyma a nodular appearance and therefore detection of a focal HCC may

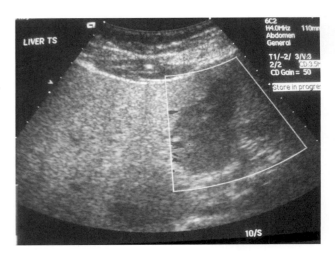

Figure 7.5 Multiple focal hepatic lesions of altered echogenicity in a patient with metastatic disease.

be more difficult in this setting. Hepatocellular carcinoma may be focal or diffuse with the latter representing a greater diagnostic challenge at sonography due to its indistinct margins. The focal lesions may be of reduced or increased reflectivity, with small lesions frequently demonstrating low echogenicity. On occasions HCC may appear as a target lesion with a hypo-echoic rim and a hyperechoic centre.

Metastases to the liver are most commonly seen in tumours arising from the colon, breast, lung, pancreas, and ovary as well as in lymphoma (Figure 7.5). Appearances may be extremely varied amongst the different tumours. The commonest pattern is that of a hypo-echoic lesion. This may be seen with tumours of any origin. Hyperechoic lesions are characteristically seen with tumours arising from the colon, pancreas, and less commonly from the kidneys and ovaries. These lesions may have a target appearance with a hypo-echoic rim.

Characterisation of focal liver lesions is often difficult on the basis of ultrasound alone. Full clinical details and results of laboratory investigations are essential. Even then further characterisation by computed tomography is usually necessary.

Portal vein thrombosis

Portal vein thrombosis may be associated with intra-abdominal sepsis, malignancy, or hypercoagulable states. At sonography echogenic thrombus may be seen within the lumen causing expansion of the vein although acutely the thrombus may be hypoechoic and even anechoic. Colour and Doppler ultrasound demonstrate lack of flow within the vein. In chronic cases a collateral circulation develops resulting in numerous serpiginous vascular channels surrounding the obliterated portal vein, a finding known as cavernous transformation of the portal vein.

Budd-Chiari syndrome

Budd-Chiari syndrome refers to the occlusion of the hepatic veins and may be associated with hypercoagulable states, haematological malignancies, or intra-abdominal malignancies such as renal cell carcinoma, adrenal carcinoma, and hepatocellular carcinoma.

Acutely, the liver is enlarged and may demonstrate patchy or generalised abnormal echogenicity. This is typically accompanied by ascites. The hepatic veins may be attenuated or may demonstrate echogenic luminal thrombus. Doppler ultrasound may show a lack of or reversal of flow within the hepatic veins. In chronic cases the liver may be generally small in size with sparing of the caudate lobe which is typically enlarged.

Ultrasound of the biliary tree

Cholelithiasis

Examination of the gallbladder should ideally be carried out after a fast to avoid errors. For detection of gallstones, the patient should be examined in the supine, right anterior oblique, and left lateral decubitus positions. The latter two positions maximise the chance of visualising a gallstone, which may be located at the gallbladder neck, by causing it to migrate to the fundus of the gallbladder. Furthermore, this helps to confirm that a focal lesion within the gallbladder is mobile and therefore likely to represent a stone.

Ultrasound is extremely sensitive in detection of gallstones and is the modality of choice for evaluation of the gallbladder. The appearance of gallstones is partly dependent on their size. Typically they are manifested as highly echogenic intraluminal foci, which cast a strong posterior acoustic shadow (Figures 7.6 and 7.7). It is essential to examine the gallbladder both on longitudinal and transverse sections to avoid mistaking gas within an adjacent loop of bowel for a gallstone.

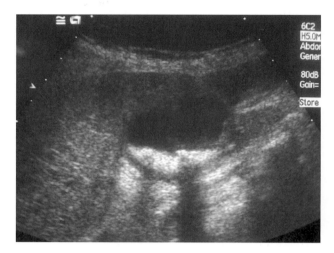

Figure 7.6 Multiple small echogenic gallstones.

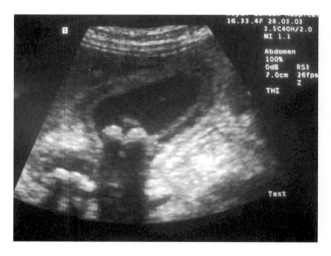

Figure 7.7 Large echogenic gallstone with posterior acoustic shadowing.

Unless impacted at the gallbladder neck, stones should be mobile, changing position in a gravity dependent manner with change in patient position as described above. Small gallstones may appear as less echogenic foci without significant posterior acoustic shadowing. These small stones may also be adherent to the gallbladder wall and therefore may not demonstrate gravity dependent motion. In such cases differentiation from a gallbladder wall polyp may be difficult.

If the gallbladder is contracted and packed with stones then normal bile may not be visualised (Figure 7.8). Gallbladder contraction may either be due to disease or due to a recent meal. In such cases appearances consist of a highly echogenic area in the gallbladder fossa with a very prominent acoustic shadow. This appearance

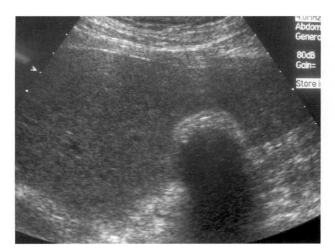

Figure 7.8 Contracted gallbladder containing stones.

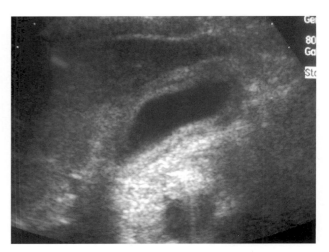

Figure 7.9 Thickened oedematous gallbladder wall with pericholecystic fluid and gallstones in a patient with acute cholecystitis.

needs to be differentiated from gas within the duodenal cap.

On occasions, layering material of lesser echogenicity may be present within the gallbladder. Such material represents sludge and is frequently seen in prolonged fasting. Such sludge may form a mass-like, mobile lesion within the gallbladder. A similar appearance may be seen in the presence of blood within the gallbladder.

Acute cholecystitis

Acute cholecystitis is associated with gallstones in the vast majority of cases. Such stones typically may be impacted in the gallbladder neck or the cystic duct resulting in a very dilated gallbladder. Classical findings in acute cholecystitis (Figure 7.9) include:

- focal tenderness over the gallbladder, elicited by exerting local pressure using the ultrasound transducer
- the presence of a thickened gallbladder wall measuring in excess of 3 mm
- oedema of the gallbladder wall, manifesting as alternating echogenic and hypo-echoic layers within the wall
- pericholecystic fluid seen as a focal anechoic fluid collection adjacent to the gallbladder, especially in the region of the fundus, reflecting a localised perforation of the wall.

The presence of gallbladder wall thickening is relatively non-specific and may be seen in a variety of other conditions. These include chronic cholecystitis, ascites of whatever cause, sepsis, acute pancreatitis, hepatitis, cirrhosis, hypo-albuminaemia, and postprandial state. More focal wall thickening may also be seen in cases with gallbladder carcinoma.

In a minority of cases clinical and sonographic features of cholecystitis may be present in the absence of gallstones. Such cases may reflect acalculus cholecystitis and are typically seen in patients with intercurrent illness.

In severe cases of cholecystitis and in particular in diabetic patients there may be development of emphysematous cholecystitis. This is reflected by presence of air within the gallbladder lumen or wall. Air within the lumen is depicted as a curvilinear non-dependent echogenic area within the gallbladder casting an acoustic shadow. This is most often seen anteriorly, obscuring visualisation of the posterior aspects of the gallbladder, and needs to be distinguished from a gallbladder packed with stones. Air within the wall causes nodular or linear echogenic foci in the substance of the wall and needs to be differentiated from a porcelain gallbladder, microabscesses in Rokitansky-Aschoff sinuses seen in gangrenous gallbladder, and adherent small stones or polyps.

Complications of acute cholecystitis include:

- perforation of the gallbladder resulting in a pericholecystic abscess
- gangrenous gallbladder demonstrating irregular asymmetric wall thickening with micro-abscesses and intraluminal septations and pseudomembranes
- empyema of the gallbladder with multiple reflective echoes within the lumen reflecting pus.

Ultrasound in obstructive jaundice

The sonographic hallmark of obstructive jaundice is intra- and extrahepatic bile duct dilatation. The bile ducts are identified as tubular structures running adjacent to the portal vein and its tributaries, without demonstrable flow on colour or Doppler ultrasound. A common bile duct (CBD) diameter of 6 mm is taken as the upper limit of normal. There is some increase in this diameter with ageing and an increase of 1 mm per decade after the age of 60 may be normal. The bile duct may also be dilated following cholecystectomy. The central hepatic bile ducts may measure up to 4 mm whilst the more peripheral intrahepatic ducts should not measure more than 40% of the diameter of the adjacent portal vein tributary. Scanning, with the patient in an oblique or decubitus position, often affords the best views of the bile ducts. Longitudinal oblique views of the porta hepatis are often the most useful.

Bile ducts in excess of the above normal diameters are indicative of biliary obstruction. Depending on the distribution of the bile duct dilatation there may be a "double barrel" appearance at the porta hepatis consisting of the dilated duct and the adjacent portal vein (Figure 7.10). With involvement of the intrahepatic ducts there is the appearance of too many tubular structures within the hepatic parenchyma (Figure 7.11).

Ultrasound is also useful in determining the level and cause of the obstruction and in guiding further investigation and management. Common causes of biliary obstruction that may be elucidated by ultrasound include the following.

Choledocholithiasis

This is illustrated as an echogenic focus, with posterior acoustic shadowing, within the dilated duct. The duct often abruptly returns to a normal calibre distal to the calculus. Mid to distal CBD stones may be difficult to visualise in the presence of gas within the duodenum and in such cases changing the position of the patient and giving oral fluids may assist in better demonstration of this region. Occasionally, there may be dilatation of the bile ducts due to sludge within the biliary tree, which is seen as less echogenic layering material in the ducts. In Mirizzi's Syndrome there is impaction of a gallstone within the cystic duct or the gallbladder

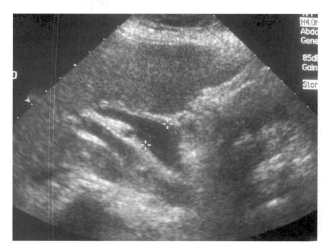

Figure 7.10   Dilated common bile duct seen anterior to the portal vein.

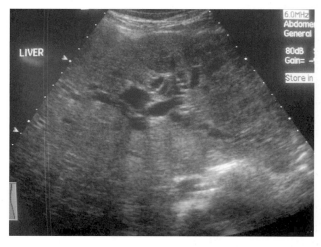

Figure 7.11   Dilated intrahepatic bile ducts adjacent to the portal vein tributaries in a patient with obstructive jaundice.

neck causing a smooth stenosis of the common hepatic duct with ensuing dilatation of the intrahepatic ducts but with a normal calibre CBD.

Pancreatic carcinoma

In such cases the CBD is dilated all the way to the head of the pancreas where a mass may be visualised. Small lesions or periampullary tumours may not be detected on ultrasound but the finding of a dilated duct extending into the head of the pancreas should be suspicious of this diagnosis. Additionally, a pancreatic head mass may cause dilatation of the pancreatic duct, resulting in a "double duct sign" illustrated as dilatation of the CBD and pancreatic ducts in the head of the pancreas.

Bile duct strictures

These may either be benign or malignant. Benign causes include previous biliary surgery, ischaemia, or strictures in the head of the pancreas secondary to chronic pancreatitis. Often in such cases a cause is not demonstrable on ultrasound. Malignant causes include cholangiocarcinoma as well as secondary tumours. Sonography may demonstrate a focal mass especially in cases of secondary tumours or lymph node involvement. However, more typically, and particularly in the presence of cholangiocarcinoma, no focal lesions or an area of diffuse thickening of the bile duct wall may be demonstrable. Isolated intrahepatic duct dilatation without a porta hepatis mass or calculi is highly suggestive of a hilar cholangiocarcinoma.

Pancreatic ultrasound

Acute pancreatitis

Acute pancreatitis is a clinical and laboratory diagnosis. The role of ultrasound in this clinical setting consists of detecting complications in particular development of fluid collections such as pseudocysts and abscesses and determining whether there are underlying predisposing factors such as calculi. However, in severe cases CT scanning may be more appropriate as it allows assessment of pancreatic enhancement and detection of necrosis, which cannot be effectively established by sonography. Ultrasound may also be used in guiding interventional procedures such as drainage of fluid collections.

The normal pancreas is iso-echoic or, with increasing age and fat deposition, hyperechoic to the liver. In pancreatitis, there is an increase in the size of the pancreas and the pancreatic parenchyma becomes more hypo-echoic due to oedema (Figure 7.12). In mild cases however, the sonographic appearances may be entirely normal. In cases of focal pancreatitis, ultrasound may demonstrate focal enlargement of the pancreas with a hypo-echoic texture simulating a pancreatic neoplasm.

With increasing severity there may be development of fluid collections in the peripancreatic and perirenal tissues and especially in the lesser sac, where fluid is seen interposed between the pancreas and the stomach. The presence of debris or gas, demonstrated as echogenic foci within a collection, is suggestive of haemorrhage or abscess formation, the latter often exhibiting a thick wall. Ultrasound is also useful in examining the vascular structures in the pancreatic bed.

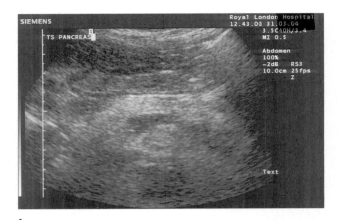

A

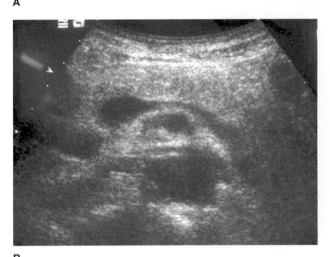

B

Figure 7.12 Oedematous and enlarged pancreas with blurred margins in acute pancreatitis. **(A)** Normal. **(B)** Acute.

Venous thrombosis, especially of the splenic and superior mesenteric veins, is evident as expansion of the vessel with intraluminal echoes and lack of colour and Doppler signal. Pseudo-aneurysm formation is characterised by a cystic lesion with an echogenic wall which possesses turbulent and disorganised flow on colour ultrasound.

Chronic pancreatitis

Chronic pancreatitis, most commonly encountered in combination with prolonged excessive alcohol intake, is sonographically identifiable as heterogeneity of the pancreatic echotexture with a combination of areas of increased echogenicity and reduced echogenicity. Superimposed on this heterogeneous background are focal areas of increased echogenicity with associated posterior acoustic shadowing consistent with calcification. The shadowing may be absent in the smaller foci of calcification.

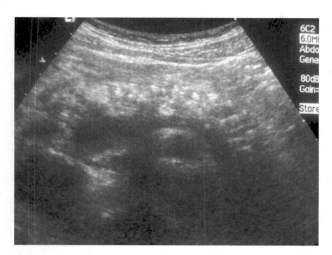

Figure 7.13 Diffuse foci of pancreatic calcification in a patient with chronic pancreatitis.

Calcification may be seen within the pancreatic parenchyma or within the pancreatic ductal system, which in addition classically display irregular dilatation (Figure 7.13). Parenchymal calcification is especially prominent in hereditary chronic calcific pancreatitis. Focal inflammatory changes may commonly occur within the pancreas resulting in a focal mass, the differentiation of which from pancreatic carcinoma may be difficult.

As with acute pancreatitis, complication such as pseudocyst formation and venous thrombosis may be evident.

Pancreatic neoplasms

Pancreatic neoplasms may be discovered incidentally, or due to their mass effect or as a result of hormone production. The latter neuroendocrine tumours may often be small and require more specialised techniques for their detection. Pancreatic head neoplasms tend to present earlier due to obstruction of the CBD causing obstructive jaundice, whilst tumours in the rest of the gland may grow to a considerable size before causing clinical symptoms.

Pancreatic carcinoma is most often hypo-echoic in nature, has a lobulated margin, and causes a focal bulge in the pancreatic contour. There may be associated dilatation of the pancreatic duct distal to the mass, seen as a tubular structure with echogenic walls and no colour flow in the substance of the gland. Lesions in the pancreatic head or the uncinate process additionally cause dilatation of the bile duct extending all the way into the head of the pancreas. Distinction from focal chronic inflammation may be difficult and may require biopsy.

Visualisation of the pancreas may be hampered by presence of gas within the stomach, duodenal loop, or the transverse colon. In such cases several manoeuvres may be helpful in allowing a more thorough examination of the pancreas. The patient may be placed in oblique, decubitus, or erect positions. Firm pressure with the ultrasound probe may help to displace a gas filled loop of bowel. Alternatively the patient can be assessed in different phases of respiration. Administration of oral fluid can result in the stomach acting as a window to enable better visualisation of the pancreatic bed. Finally the tail of the pancreas may be better examined at the splenic hilum by scanning through the left upper quadrant and using the spleen as a sonographic window.

Renal ultrasound

Renal tract calculi

Stone disease is a very common cause of presentation to the accident and emergency department. A number of modalities and investigations may be used in demonstration of calculi. These include plain films, tomography, intravenous urogram (IVU), ultrasound, and CT.

The sensitivity of ultrasound is dependent on the location and size of the calculus, being highest for detection of renal and lower ureteric calculi. Demonstration of upper and mid-ureteric calculi may be hampered by the presence of bowel gas and such stones may be easily missed on ultrasound especially if the ureter is not dilated. Furthermore, even in the presence of obstruction pelvicalyceal and ureteric dilatation may be absent acutely.

Calculi are seen as highly echogenic foci casting a well defined and intense acoustic shadow (Figure 7.14). Calculi smaller than 5 mm may be very difficult to demonstrate and may not exhibit acoustic shadowing. To maximise the chances of visualisation of calculi the patient should be examined from varying angles and in different positions using the highest frequency transducer possible. Reducing the gain and using tissue harmonics accentuates the characteristics of the stone. The patient should be examined with a moderately full bladder as the bladder will then act as an acoustic window through which the distal ureters may be visualised. If dilated these will be seen as anechoic tubular structures posterior to the bladder. Differentiation from vessels can be made using Doppler.

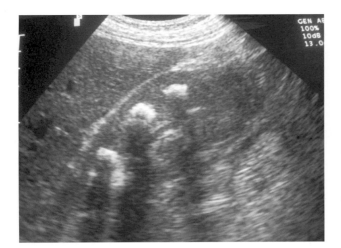

A

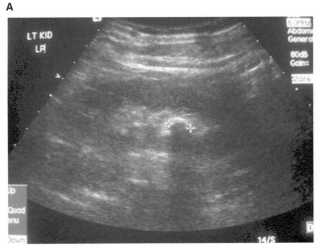

B

Figure 7.14 Echogenic intra-renal focus with posterior acoustic shadowing consistent with a renal calculus. **(A)** Multiple stones. **(B)** Single renal calculus (calipers).

Occasionally, other entities may mimic renal calculi on ultrasound. These include the normal renal sinus fat, renal artery calcification, and intrarenal gas. The sinus fat, although echogenic, especially if tissue harmonics is employed, does not tend to produce acoustic shadowing. Renal artery calcification tends to produce linear echogenic bands whilst the shadowing associated with intrarenal gas is not as well defined.

Renal tract obstruction

The hallmark of renal tract obstruction on ultrasound is collecting system dilatation. However, obstruction may occur without significant collecting system dilatation especially if it is acute, and conversely pelvicalyceal dilatation may be seen in the absence of obstruction typically in the setting of reflux.

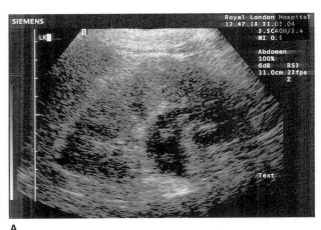

A

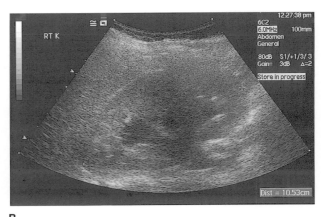

B

Figure 7.15 Communicating central fluid collections consistent with pelvicalyceal dilatation in a patient with renal tract obstruction. **(A)** Hydronephrosis **(B)** Gross hydronephrosis.

Pelvicalyceal dilatation is seen as central anechoic fluid collections within the kidneys. Differentiation from renal cysts requires demonstration of communication between the various components of the fluid collection (Figure 7.15). The dilated renal pelvis is typically seen medially surrounded by the echogenic sinus fat. The dilated calyces are likewise surrounded by sinus fat but can be shown to communicate with the renal pelvis. More distally the dilated renal pelvis may be seen to communicate with a dilated proximal ureter, illustrated as an anechoic tubular structure lying anterior to the psoas muscles. The mid-ureter is typically the hardest segment to visualise, being commonly obscured by bowel gas. The dilated distal ureters may be seen as tubular structures posterior to the bladder.

Furthermore, ultrasound may also be used to elucidate the cause of obstruction such as renal calculi, retroperitoneal, and pelvic masses, as well as the level of the obstruction.

Pyonephrosis

Pyonephrosis occurs as a result of infection of an obstructed system. Classically this is manifested as a dilated collecting system containing echoes and debris, which may demonstrate layering or may be seen to move with a change in the patient position. However, the presence of low level echoes and debris is not invariable and conversely echoes may be seen in a dilated pelvicalyceal system as a result of haemorrhage. In such cases ultrasound guided aspiration may be required. In severe cases gas may be seen in the collecting system.

Pyelonephritis

Pyelonephritis is most commonly secondary to an ascending infection but may on occasions be due to haematogenous spread. Ultrasound is not usually required in the acute setting but should be performed if there is no improvement in clinical, haematological, or biochemical markers despite adequate treatment in order to detect abscess development or obstruction. In uncomplicated cases ultrasound should be carried out once the acute episode has resolved in order to determine whether there are any underlying structural abnormalities predisposing to pyelonephritis.

In the acute setting, renal ultrasound may be normal. In abnormal cases, the kidney may be enlarged with loss of the normal corticomedullary differentiation. The renal parenchyma may be hypo-echoic due to oedema or hyperechoic if there is haemorrhagic change.

Renal abscess

In the presence of severe infection or with delayed treatment of infections, a renal abscess may develop. Renal abscesses may be unilocular or multilocular. Mutilocular collections may coalesce to form a larger collection. These are generally hypo-echoic with posterior acoustic enhancement. On some occasions they may be completely anechoic or rarely hyperechoic due to the presence of gas within the abscess. Small abscesses may respond to intravenous antibiotic therapy but larger collections generally require percutaneous drainage.

Renal trauma

Computed tomography is the modality of choice in renal trauma and ultrasound has no role in the acute setting. The only role for ultrasound would be in follow-up of perirenal collections.

Splenic ultrasound

The spleen is best visualised via an intercostal approach with the transducer parallel to the ribs. This may be carried out in the supine or the left anterior oblique position. The spleen is said to be enlarged if it measures more than 12 cm from the upper pole to the lower pole. Splenic enlargement may be seen in lymphoproliferative and myelo-proliferative disorders, portal hypertension and cirrhosis, infections such as infectious mono-nucleosis, AIDS and malaria, and in a variety of other disorders such as connective tissue disease and sarcoidosis. Splenomegaly may also be seen in portal vein and splenic vein thrombosis and therefore assessment of the portal and splenic veins by Doppler sonography is important. Splenomegaly is not invariable in many of the above conditions.

Focal splenic lesions may be visualised in splenic cysts, haemangiomas, splenic abscesses, infarcts, lymphoma, and metastatic disease. The clinical detail is often essential in distinguishing between these lesions. Metastatic involvement is most common with melanoma, bronchogenic, ovarian, and breast carcinoma.

The spleen is the most commonly injured organ in blunt abdominal trauma. Computed tomography is the modality of choice in detection and characterisation of splenic injuries. However, ultrasound may demonstrate abnormalities associated with splenic traumatic injury. These include free fluid, which may be located in the left subphrenic space or in the rest of the abdomen or pelvis, fluid attenuation extending into the splenic parenchyma, or a heterogeneous echotexture to the splenic parenchyma reflecting intraparenchymal haemorrhage.

The appendix

Effective sonographic evaluation of the appendix requires a high frequency transducer (7 MHz or above). Using the transducer, progressively increased pressure is applied in the right iliac fossa, to displace bowel gas and contents. This technique is known as graded compression.

The normal appendix may be identified as a blind ending tubular structure with a diameter of less than 7 mm. In acute appendicitis there is

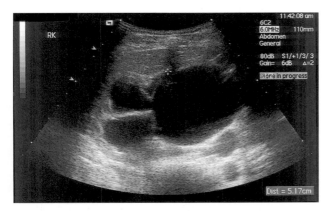

Figure 7.16 A dilated non-compressible appendix in acute appendicitis.

focal tenderness over the appendix, the diameter is enlarged to greater than 9 mm and the wall has a multilayered appearance. In addition the distended lumen is not compressible by applying further pressure with the probe (Figure 7.16). In some cases a calcified intraluminal appendicolith may be visualised. An area of increased reflectivity surrounding the appendix and a small amount of free fluid indicate adjacent inflammatory changes in the mesentery. Inflammation of tissues also results in increased vascularity of the appendix and the surrounding tissues on colour ultrasound.

If there has been a delay in diagnosis, an appendiceal abscess may develop. This is reflected by the presence of a fluid collection in the right iliac fossa with inflammatory change in the surrounding mesentery illustrated by increased echogenicity of the fat. In some cases there may be an inflammatory mass caused by matting of loops of bowel and adjacent inflammation. This causes an ill-defined hypo-echoic mass lesion with surrounding inflammation. In the presence of an abscess, ultrasound may be used for placement of a percutaneous drain.

Aortic aneurysms

Ultrasound is an effective and quick method to determine the presence of an aneurysm. Visualisation of the aorta may be hampered by the presence of bowel gas. However, usually the entire aorta may be adequately examined by using an anterior approach combined with further views from the flanks. Measurement of aneurysm size should be undertaken on transverse and longitudinal scans from the outer wall to outer wall of the aneurysm.

The aneurysm normally has an echogenic wall especially in the presence of calcification. The lumen is of very low echogenicity and demonstrates flow on colour scanning. There is usually mural thrombus present, depicted as a semilunar hypo-echoic area between the wall and the lumen.

Ultrasound may be used to assess the size of the aneurysm, its relationship to the renal arteries by using colour flow to illustrate the vessels and its relationship to the aortic bifurcation. Its extent can be assessed on the longitudinal scans.

The hallmark of a leaking aneurysm is that of retroperitoneal haematoma. This is characterised by a very ill-defined heterogeneous but predominantly hyperechoic area in the retroperitoneum. Its detection may be difficult as it is rather poorly marginated and blends into surrounding structures. Secondary signs include anterior displacement of the kidneys and the presence of free fluid.

Summary

This chapter has described the ultrasound findings associated with a variety of acute abdominal conditions that may present to the emergency department. The non-radiologist must continue to use ultrasound to answer focussed questions in the emergency evaluation of abdominal conditions (for example, is the right upper quadrant pain cholecystitis?) and must be aware that any imaging modality is only an adjunct to a full history and clinical examination.

8 Bedside ultrasound as an adjunct in the evaluation of critically ill patients

ANTHONY J DEAN

Objectives
- To introduce the concept of emergency medicine bedside ultrasound
- To discuss ultrasound diagnosis of acute medical conditions
- To describe the technique for ultrasound evaluation of unexplained hypotension and shortness of breath

Introduction

While the utility of ultrasound in the management of blunt trauma is well established, the majority of patients with respiratory or circulatory insufficiency encountered in emergency practice are more likely to have a non-traumatic aetiology for their disease. Cardiac tamponade, pulmonary embolus, or acute abdominal aortic aneurysm are causes of hypotension no less lethal than trauma, affording "golden minutes" rather than a "golden hour" for life saving intervention. Such patients are usually too sick to provide a clear or detailed history, and the diagnostic evaluation is, of necessity, limited and focussed. In cardio-pulmonary arrest (CPA) the final, pre-mortal phase of evaluation of respiratory and circulatory instability is further telescoped, and proceeds concomitantly with treatment according to the time-honoured priorities of "Airway, Breathing, Circulation". With such critically ill patients, a device that could diagnose several causes of undifferentiated respiratory or circulatory compromise, evaluate the results of therapeutic interventions, and be deployed at the bedside by the treating physician within seconds of a patient's arrival, would obviously be of great value. Ultrasonography is such a modality.

With ongoing technological advances that allow higher resolution images on more affordable, mobile, and user-friendly equipment, a growing body of literature describes the use of bedside ultrasound in this setting. As has been noted by surgical sonographers with respect to their use of ultrasound in the evaluation of trauma, no specialty "has ownership of technology".[1] This position is supported by the American Medical Association, which has mandated that "standards ... [for the use of ultrasound be] ... developed by each physician's respective specialty society".[2] The acronym "EMBU" (Emergency Medicine Bedside Ultrasound), used throughout this chapter, emphasises key elements of sonography as practised by emergency physicians. It is conducted by the *treating clinician at the bedside* as an integrated component of the management of *emergency* conditions. This chapter will describe the evolving efforts of practitioners to appropriate, adapt, and integrate a variety of sonographic techniques in order to improve the care of the critically ill.

EMBU: case histories

The following cases illustrate some representative emergency scenarios. Several other examples have been published in articles exploring this topic.[3,4]

Case 1

A 25-year-old female was brought to the emergency department (ED) by fire rescue for an "asthma attack". Medics reported that the family "had heard a crash", but the patient had denied trauma, and complained only of shortness of breath. On arrival the patient denied underlying medical problems, including heart disease, lung disease, pregnancy, or drug use. The patient was agitated and diaphoretic with a heart rate (HR) of 140, blood pressure (BP) 100/60, respiratory rate (RR) 36, and oxygen saturation 100%. The breath sounds were symmetrical and clear. Abdominal exam was remarkable for what appeared to be a gravid fundus, with closed os on pelvic examination. There was no sign of vaginal blood or trauma. The patient's

---

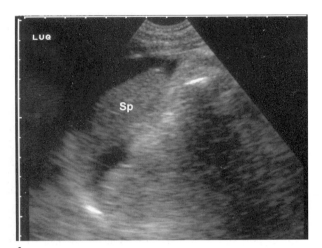

A

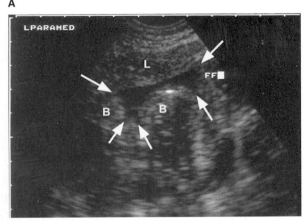

B

Figure 8.1 (A) A left upper quadrant view showing the spleen (Sp) surrounded by hypo-echoic (black on the image) blood. Unclotted blood below the liver margin (L) surrounding bowel **(B)** in the right hypochondrium demonstrates the characteristic "pointy" morphology (arrows) of pathologic fluid as it flows between the "roundy" shapes of normal intra-abdominal organs. Morison's Pouch, not seen in this view, was distended with fluid.

condition deteriorated rapidly over the following minutes, with her systolic BP falling to 60 mmHg despite aggressive fluid resuscitation. EMBU was performed, showing extensive intraperitoneal fluid with an apparently viable intrauterine pregnancy (IUP) (Figures 8.1A and 8.1B). As a result of these findings, the patient was rushed to the operating room less than 20 minutes after her arrival, where a ruptured uterus was identified and hysterectomy was performed. After a complicated course, the patient left the hospital completely recovered 21 days later.

Case 2

A 55-year-old female presented with two days' shortness of breath, with associated substernal and epigastric pain. The patient was well known to the ED for recurrent bouts of pancreatitis associated with ongoing heavy alcohol consumption, and emphysema with continued heavy tobacco use. The patient was in obvious distress, anxious, agitated, and gasping for breath. Her HR was 130, RR 30, and BP 110/60, with oxygen saturation of 97% on room air. Her lung sounds were distant but clear bilaterally. Examination was otherwise unremarkable except for jugular venous distension, and epigastric tenderness. The cardiology service was consulted for urgent echocardiography to exclude pericardial tamponade. The cardiologist stated that the patient did not require urgent echocardiography because her symptoms could be explained by her known pancreatitis and restrictive lung disease. In view of the continued suspicion of tamponade, a junior house officer performed EMBU, identifying a massive pericardial effusion with tamponade (Figure 8.2). Urgent pericardiotomy drained 1400 cc of sanguineous pericardial fluid, subsequently identified as being due to metastatic adenocarcinoma of the lung.

Case 3

A 24-year-old female fainted while walking to the bathroom at home at around 7 am. She complained of poorly defined pelvic pain and right upper quadrant discomfort. The patient had no significant past medical history. Her last normal menstrual period was two weeks ago. Vital signs were as follows: afebrile, HR 90, RR 16, BP 100/60, with orthostatic tachycardia and dizziness on standing. Her physical examination was otherwise normal except for mild right upper quadrant and suprapubic tenderness with mild right adnexal tenderness on pelvic examination. The diagnostic work-up was unrevealing, with normal ECG, blood indices, electrolytes, and negative pregnancy test. Despite 2 litres of normal saline intravenously, the BP dropped to the 80s, with dizziness while supine. EMBU evaluation for peritoneal, pleural, and pericardial fluid revealed a large quantity of free fluid and clot in the pelvis, left upper quadrant, and Morison's pouch (Figures 8.3A, B, and C), with identification of a large, partially collapsed right ovarian cyst. The patient was managed conservatively despite a haemoglobin that dropped to 8. She was discharged two days later with the diagnosis of ruptured haemorrhagic ovarian cyst.

Ultrasound in the evaluation of unexplained hypotension

Critically ill patients, whether they be surgical or medical, have the common characteristic of

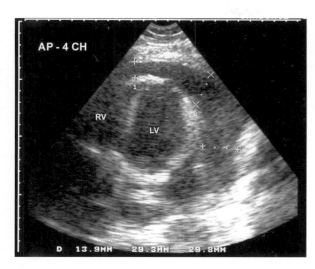

Figure 8.2 Large circumferential pericardial effusion (between callipers) which is in excess of 3 cm in thickness in some areas (LV = left ventricle, RV = right ventricle).

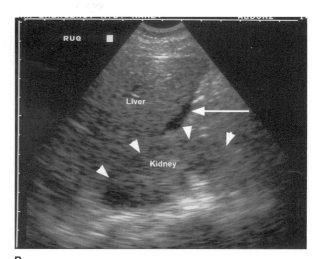

B

Figure 8.3(B) In this sagittal view of the right upper quadrant, the margin of the kidney is highlighted with arrowheads. Morison's pouch, the potential space between the liver and kidney, is filling with free fluid: the hypo-echoic area

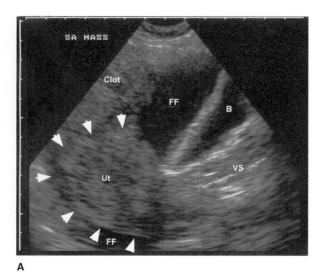

A

Figure 8.3(A) Midline sagittal view of the pelvis showing free fluid (FF) and clot surrounding the uterus (arrowheads), superior and anterior to the bladder (B). The vaginal stripe (VS) can be seen behind the bladder.

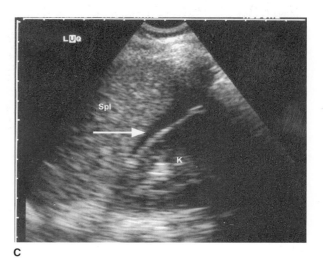

C

Figure 8.3(C) In the left upper quadrant the potential space between the spleen (Spl) and kidney (K) is filling with free fluid with its characteristically "pointy" shape (tip of arrow).

Case 4

A 52-year-old male presented complaining of sudden onset of severe mid-sternal chest pain about 30 minutes earlier, with nausea, diaphoresis, and shortness of breath. The patient had not seen a doctor since childhood. On physical examination the patient was in discomfort and diaphoretic with a BP of 110/62 (equal in both arms), a HR of 52, a RR of 22, and normal oxygen saturation. An ECG showed sinus bradycardia with frequent premature nodal beats, ventricular hypertrophy, and nonspecific ST segment abnormalities. An EMBU showed a large pericardial effusion without tamponade

(Figure 8.4A). In addition, on high parasternal long axis views, a mobile flap in the aortic root can faintly be seen, and in abdominal views of the descending aorta colour-flow Doppler reveals a pseudolumen surrounded by occluded aorta (Figure 8.4B). The cardiothoracic surgery service was consulted within minutes of the patient's arrival. He was expeditiously taken to the operating room for urgent repair of his acute aortic dissection.

benefiting from immediate evaluation and treatment without removal from the resuscitation area. However, in contrast to the setting of trauma,

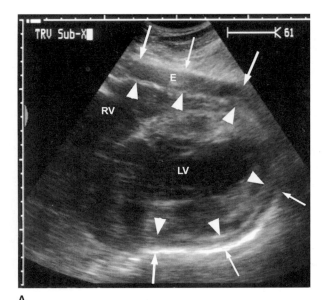

A

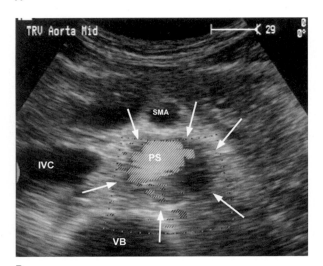

B

Figure 8.4 **(A)** Subxiphoid view showing the fluid in the highly echogenic pericardium (arrows) and less echogenic epicardium (arrowheads), defining the fluid filled pericardial sac. Echoes (E) within the pericardial effusion are suggestive of freshly clotted blood (RV = right ventricle, LV = left ventricle). **(B)** A transverse view of the aorta (arrows) at the level of the superior mesenteric artery (SMA) reveals a normal sized aorta with flow limited to a pseudolumen (PS) as demonstrated by colour-flow Doppler. (IVC = inferior vena cava; VB = vertebral body).

many of the sonographic diagnoses in critically ill "medical" patients go beyond the mere identification of abnormal collections of "free fluid". While this extends the diagnostic utility of bedside sonography, it makes it technically more challenging. Emergency sonographers can surmount these challenges with relative ease for several reasons.

Case 5

A 68-year-old woman with a history of hypertension and atrial fibrillation presented to the ED in cardiac arrest. Earlier, the patient had complained of groin pain, and about 20 minutes prior to arrival she had collapsed. On arrival, she was intubated, pulseless, with a bradycardic narrow complex rhythm on the cardiac monitor. While cardiopulmonary resuscitation was ongoing, an EMBU was performed. The subxiphoid view of the heart showed weak coordinated cardiac motion with complete valve closure. Sonographic evaluation of the abdominal area revealed an 8.1 cm abdominal aortic aneurysm (AAA) with extraluminal clot (Figure 8.5). Intraperitoneal fluid was not seen. Vascular surgeons were consulted urgently. Within 30 minutes of her arrival, the patient was transported to the operating room, where she later expired.

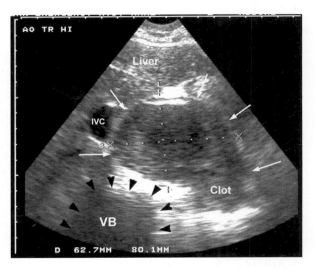

Figure 8.5 To avoid mistaking other structures for the aorta, it is often helpful for the sonologist to start by identifying the vertebral body (VB): a round structure with posterior shadowing (arrowheads). The aorta (arrows) appears to have an irregular shape due to the presence of extraluminal clot. In most cases of abdominal aortic aneurysm the liver does not provide a sonographic window, as it does here. This patient's aneurysm was indeed found to be both thoracic and abdominal.

- First, many of the sonographic techniques are familiar from other bedside applications.
- Second, as diseases progress to the point of causing haemodynamic instability, they give rise to increasingly gross sonographic findings.
- Third, while specialists such as echocardiologists have more extensive training and experience, a more focussed area of expertise, access to higher resolution equipment, and the luxury of more time in the examination of generally stable patients, all of which allow for more technical

quantitative analyses, several clinically important parameters in the critically ill can be effectively evaluated in qualitative terms.

Examples of such information obtained by bedside echocardiography of critically ill patients would include qualitative determinations of ejection fraction, relative ventricular size, adequacy of cardiac filling, and presence or absence of cardiac motion. This is borne out by investigations showing the utility of echocardiography by cardiologists using limited protocols and hand-held ultrasound devices to perform focussed qualitative evaluations.[5–7]

Body regions to be investigated and sonographic findings to be sought by EMBU in the evaluation of unexplained hypotension, PEA or cardiopulmonary arrest. (# indicates conditions which can be identified, but cannot be reliably excluded with EMBU.)

EMBU of the thorax

Evaluation of the pericardium
    Effusion +/−tamponade
Evaluation of the heart
    Empty hyperdynamic heart
    Global wall motion abnormalities
    Focal wall motion abnormalities #
    Sonographic findings of pulmonary embolus (see text) #
    Sonographic findings of right-sided MI (see text) #
    Gross dynamic or structural abnormalities of the heart valves #
Evaluation of the proximal aorta
    Mobile intimal flap #
Evaluation of the pleural spaces
    Sonographic findings of pneumothorax (see text)
    Massive pleural effusion
    Massive pulmonary consolidation

EMBU of the abdomen

Inferior vena cava*
    Evaluation of size, collapse index (see text)
    Identification of intraluminal clot or other obstruction
Abdominal aorta
    Aortic diameter
    Intimal flap, pseudolumen
Peritoneal cavity
    Free fluid
    Sonographic findings of pneumoperitoneum (see text)

Lower extremity limited compression ultrasonography

*The IVC is usually examined in the subxiphoid window concurrently with the evaluation of the thorax.

Regions that may need sonographic assessment in the evaluation of a patient with unexplained hypotension are listed above, including the thorax, the aorta, the body cavities (peritoneal and pleural), and the deep veins of the lower extremities. As with all tests used in emergency practice, the sonographic evaluation will be directed by, and interpreted in the context of, the patient's entire clinical picture. In the absence of clinical clues, a methodical sequential approach may be necessary, and a variety of such protocols has been reported.[3,4,8] More commonly, there is some rudimentary information to direct and prioritise the sonographic evaluation. For example, a patient who had complained of abdominal pain prior to a syncopal event might have the aorta and peritoneal spaces examined first (as in Cases 3 and 5), although such an approach would initially miss the tamponade in Case 2. Conversely, a patient with a history of cancer and distended neck veins would probably prompt initial evaluation for cardiac tamponade and pulmonary embolus. Table 8.1 lists the sonographic findings and their clinical significance in assessing various regions of the body. The present discussion will focus on those not described in detail elsewhere in this text.

Pericardial effusion and tamponade

Clinically significant pericardial effusion and tamponade are described in the chapters on trauma. It should be noted that Beck's triad is a late finding in tamponade, and it would certainly benefit the patient to have this diagnosis made prior to the onset of hypotension. It is likely that, with more widespread utilisation of EMBU, tamponade will be increasingly identified prior to onset of haemodynamic compromise. The identification of pericardial effusion or tamponade in the setting of chest pain may be due to aortic dissection or ventricular free wall rupture. The distinction between these may be difficult on clinical, electrocardiographic, or sonographic grounds. The presence of an intimal flap in the ascending or descending aorta (see Case 4 and Figure 8.4B), or the identification of a defect in the ventricular wall may clarify the matter. Positional pleuritic chest pain, repetitive unprovoked vomiting, and restlessness or agitation are suggestive of ventricular free wall rupture. In either case, the assistance of a cardiothoracic surgeon is urgently needed.

Table 8.1 **Clinical significance of various sonographic findings in assessment of severe dyspnoea, hypotension, and during cardiopulmonary resuscitation**

Organ of interest and sonographic finding	*Clinical significance*
Heart and mediastinum	
Pericardial effusion +/– right atrial or ventricular collapse during diastole	Pericardial effusion +/– tamponade. Consider acute ventricular rupture, aortic dissection
Small hyperdynamic heart, end-systolic ventricular collapse	Intravascular hypovolaemia
Well filled hyperdynamic heart	Peripheral vasodilation: consider sepsis, anaphylaxis, vasodilators
Well filled dynamic heart with decreased ejection fraction	Consider sepsis, end-stage cardiomyopathy, metabolic, or ischaemic causes
Dilated RV, +/– paradoxical septal motion, +/– RV hypokinesis, +/– intracardiac thrombus, tricuspid regurgitation	Massive pulmonary embolus
Dilated RV, +/– paradoxical septal motion, +/– RV hypokinesis, no tricuspid regurgitation	RV infarct
Decrease or absence of myocardial wall motion; absence of valve closure, valve motion; presence of intracardiac gel-like densities	Each represents progressive cardiac dysfunction in PEA. Consider ischaemic, toxic, metabolic causes
Focal wall motion abnormalities	Acute coronary syndrome
Difficulty identifying the heart on all views	Consider tension pneumothorax
Marked displacement of heart in subxiphoid view to left or right	Right or left tension pneumothorax (respectively)
Intimal flap on high PSLA or suprasternal views	Aortic dissection
Gross dynamic or structural abnormalities of the heart valves	Papillary muscle rupture, valvular lesions
Abdomen	
Intraperitoneal free fluid	Hemoperitoneum *v* ascites
Aorta for AAA and intimal flap	Acute AAA, aortic dissection
IVC collapse	Intravascular hypovolaemia
IVC distended absence of normal respiratory variation	Consider pulmonary embolus, acute RV infarct, acute right sided heart failure
Absence of normal sliding of parietal-visceral peritoneum interface, linear reverberation artefacts	Pneumoperitoneum
Pleural spaces	
Pleural free fluid +/– internal echodensities	Pleural effusion; if internal echodensities: consider empyema *v* clotted blood
Absence of "pleural sliding" sign	Pneumothorax
Multiple comet tail artefacts	Consider "wet lungs": CHF, ARDS, etc
Ultrasound through transmission of lung	Pulmonary consolidation
Lower extremities	
Non-compressible common femoral and/or popliteal veins	DVT

Abbreviations: AAA: abdominal aortic aneurysm; ARDS: adult respiratory distress syndrome; CHF: congestive heart failure; DVT: deep venous thrombosis; IVC: inferior vena cava; PEA: pulseless electrical activity; PSLA: parasternal long axis; RV: right ventricle

Shock states and causes of global myocardial dysfunction

If tamponade is excluded, the heart and cardiac chambers should be evaluated for gross abnormalities of size and motion. A hyperdynamic heart with near or complete end-systolic collapse should prompt a clinical and sonographic search for a cause of acute hypovolaemia. The sonographic evaluation will focus on the major body cavities for evidence of abnormal fluid collections. The potential spaces that need to be examined for free fluid are listed below and in Figure 8.6.

Regions and potential spaces to be evaluated in the search for pathological fluid collections

Right costal and subcostal region, midclavicular to posterior axillary line (from superior to inferior)
    Pleural space
    Subphrenic space
    Morison's pouch
    Right colic gutter/inferior pole of right kidney
Subxiphoid
    Pericardial space
Left costal and subcostal region, midclavicular to posterior axillary line (from superior to inferior)
    Left pleural space
    Subphrenic space
    Splenorenal space
    Left colic gutter/inferior pole of left kidney
Suprapubic
    Pouch of Douglas/rectouterine space

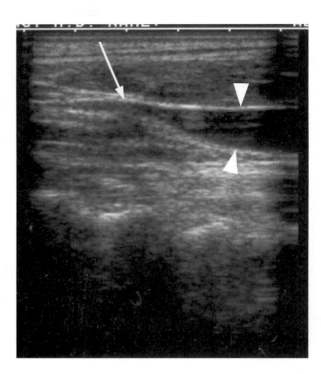

Figure 8.7 In a longitudinal view, the fluid column of blood within the internal jugular vein (between arrowheads) resembles the neck of a wine bottle. The apex of the fluid column (arrow) should be marked at the end of expiration. Five centimetres are added to the vertical distance of this point from the sternal angle to compute right sided central venous pressure (see text). Measurements may be more accurate scanning in a transverse plane.

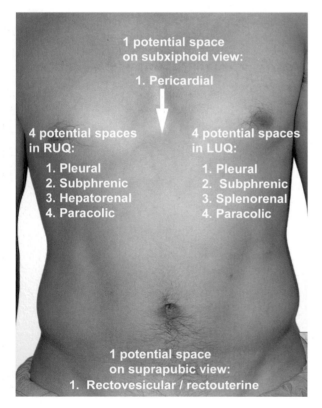

Figure 8.6 Potential spaces to be checked for occult fluid collections. Compare with the text box listing the potential spaces to be evaluated.

The same sonographic windows and methodical approach are used as in the trauma examination. An estimation of the intravascular volume status can also be made by evaluation of the inferior vena cava (IVC). While the accuracy of this technique is not perfect in stable patients, caval collapse in unexplained hypotension strongly suggests intravascular volume depletion. The interpretation of sonographically identified IVC distension is considered below, in the discussion of pulmonary embolus.

Sonographic assessment of the internal jugular vein can also be used to measure central venous pressure.[9] With the patient supine, the internal jugular vein is identified in longitudinal section, and the patient elevated to the point at which the vein can be seen tapering to a point of collapse (see Figure 8.7). At this point, the vein has the appearance of the neck of a wine bottle, thick inferiorly, and tapering in a cephalad direction. The superior extent of the jugular venous column will be seen to undulate with respirations and cardiac contraction. The examiner must be careful to maintain light contact with the skin or the vein will collapse from pressure applied by the transducer. The vertical height from the point of complete collapse to the sternal angle of Louis is added to 5 cm for a measure of central venous pressure. If the vein is not distended with the patient supine, central venous pressure is extremely low: a diagnosis that could be corroborated by cardiac findings as described above.

In the absence of findings of intravascular volume depletion, the echocardiographic evaluation continues with a qualitative assessment of the cardiac chambers and cardiac wall motion. A well-filled heart that is hyperdynamic suggests distributive shock due to sepsis, anaphylaxis, or vasodilator toxicity. A large heart with global hypokinesis can be due to ischaemic, metabolic, toxicologic, or septic causes (see the discussion of pulseless electrical activity, below). Isolated right ventricular abnormalities are considered below. While the assessment of focal wall motion abnormalities in stable patients with chest pain is beyond the skill of most emergency sonologists, the gross derangements sufficiently profound to cause cardiogenic shock are likely to be more easily identifiable.[10] This has been confirmed by a study that showed emergency physicians to be as accurate as cardiologists in the recognition of systolic dysfunction in hypotensive patients.[8] This approach is also supported by the finding that while a variety of relatively arcane parameters have been used to measure ejection fraction, gross visual estimates are reliable, and possibly no less accurate.[11–13] One study demonstrated the ability of second and third year internal medicine residents with one hour's training to perform adequate sonographic examinations of left ventricular function using a hand-held device. They also attained significant improvement of diagnostic accuracy in distinguishing asymptomatic patients with and without left ventricular dysfunction.[7] To hone the ability of identifying qualitative abnormalities in the critically ill, emergency physicians should consciously study the sonographic appearance of the heart during evaluations of patients with normal cardiac function.

Pulmonary embolus and right ventricular infarction

Studies investigating the accuracy of echocardiography in the diagnosis of pulmonary embolus (PE) in stable patients have conflicting results, so that its utility in the routine work-up of PE is controversial.[14] However, similar to myocardial ischemia with shock, PE sufficient to cause haemodynamic instability results in gross, readily identifiable, echocardiographic abnormalities.[15,16] Several qualitative B- and

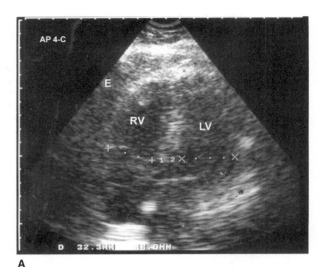

A

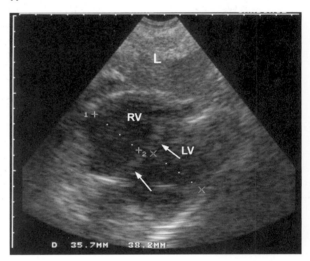

B

Figure 8.8 Sonographic signs in pulmonary embolus. The maximum normal RV end diastolic dimension (EDD) is < 27 mm. The normal RV to LV EDD ratio is < 60% (see text). **(A)** An apical four-chamber view shows the right ventricle (RV) with an EDD of 32 mm, while that of the left ventricle (LV) is 38 mm. **(B)** The image of the heart using the liver (L) as a sonographic window identifies this as a subxiphoid view. There is an increased RV to LV EDD ratio of 93%, with enlargement of the RV and abnormal bulging of the septum towards the left ventricle (arrows).

M-mode parameters can easily be assessed by the emergency echocardiographer in the evaluation of massive PE, including right to left ventricular dimension ratio, intracardiac thrombus, septal wall flattening, abnormal septal wall motion, and loss of the normal inferior vena cava (IVC) collapse index.[17–19] These are discussed in detail below. Other sonographic findings, such as tricuspid regurgitation peak velocities and pulmonary artery hypertension, require colour-flow and spectral Doppler analysis. These are techniques, at this

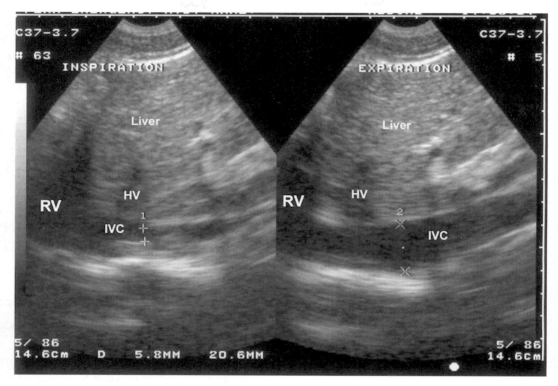

Figure 8.9 A normal collapse index of > 40%. Longitudinal views of the inferior vena cava (IVC, between callipers) on inspiration (left image) and expiration (right image) immediately below the hepatic veins (HV) show diameters of 5·8 and 20·6 mm respectively, in this patient without pulmonary embolus (see text and text box). Note that it is possible to measure the IVC either longitudinally or transversely, but that both methods may present challenges to the sonographer. In the longitudinal view errors arise if the plane of the ultrasound moves from the centre of the IVC. In the transverse plane, diaphragmatic excursion may impede accurate measurement, although this method is usually easier and more accurate.

time, beyond the expertise of most emergency medicine bedside sonographers.[15]

The normal right ventricular (RV) end-diastolic dimension, measured at the tips of the tricuspid leaflets in the apical 4-chamber view (or subxiphoid, if that is not possible) should be less than 27 mm.[19] In PE, the RV will exceed this size (Figures 8.8A and 8.8B). Another measure of RV dilation which is sometimes easier to obtain by a qualitative visual estimate without the need for freezing images and using callipers, is the end-diastolic right to left ventricular ratio, which is normally < 60% (Figure 8.8). In patients with acute PE, the ratio is almost always > 100%. Chronic pulmonary hypertension also causes RV dilation, but will be accompanied by a thickened, vigorously contracting ventricular wall, whereas in PE the RV wall is effaced (< 7 mm). RV infarct and PE may cause similar clinical, haemodynamic, and sonographic findings, making distinction difficult. Ventricular distension with a thin, hypokinetic RV free wall, septal flattening, and paradoxical septal motion, defined by abnormal contraction of the septal wall towards the RV lumen in systole, and relaxation of the wall towards the left ventricle in diastole, are all seen in both massive PE, and RV infarct.[15,20] Often the distinction can be made electrocardiographically; if not, the two can be relatively easily differentiated by the presence or absence of tricuspid regurgitation (TR) if an ultrasound machine with colour-flow Doppler capability is available. In one series of 60 patients with acute PE, TR occurred in 99%, and its presence distinguishes the high pressure overload state of acute PE from the low pressure overload state of RV infarction in which TR is uncommon.[19]

Another marker of PE is the inferior vena caval (IVC) collapse index. The IVC collapse index is defined as the difference between the IVC diameter in forced inspiration ("sniff") and its diameter in forced expiration, divided by its diameter in forced expiration (see below, and figure 8.9).

Inferior vena caval (IVC) collapse index

$$\text{IVC collapse index} = \frac{[\text{IVCD on expiration} - \text{IVCD on inspiration}]}{\text{IVCD on expiration}}$$

The IVC collapse index is normally > 40%.

For example, in the patient shown in Figure 8.9:

$$\text{IVC collapse index} = \frac{[20\cdot6 - 5\cdot8]}{20\cdot6} = 71\cdot8\%$$

IVCD = IVC diameter.
Note all measurements made in diastole

Measurements are made just inferior to the junction of the hepatic veins on the subxiphoid view, and should be made in diastole. A normal index is > 40%, and is likely to be less in cases of significant right ventricular failure. Studies have used these sonographic findings singly, or in combination to identify PE with a wide range of results.[15–17,21] As is often the case in EMBU, data to make absolute rules are lacking, and sonographic findings will need to be integrated with the entire clinical picture to determine their significance.

Acute dissection of the aorta

The most accurate sonographic method of diagnosis of aortic dissection is transoesophageal echocardiography (TEE). If this technology is not immediately available, this diagnosis can also be made by the transthoracic approach (TTE), as occurred in Case 4. The latter is 80% sensitive and 93% specific in the diagnosis of type A (proximal) aortic dissection, so that while this technique may not be sufficiently sensitive to exclude the diagnosis, there is no reason why it should not be used in the attempt to rule it in. The characteristic finding of a delicate fluttering echodensity in the aortic lumen should be sought in high parasternal, long axis views of the aortic root, and in the suprasternal window. The latter is obtained by placing a small footprint transducer in the suprasternal notch and angling it sharply inferiorly (usually about 150 degrees from the plane of the sternum). Since the aortic arch runs from an anterior right-sided to a posterior left-sided location, the plane of the probe is rotated clockwise approximately 30 degrees (between "1 and 2 o'clock") to obtain a longitudinal view of

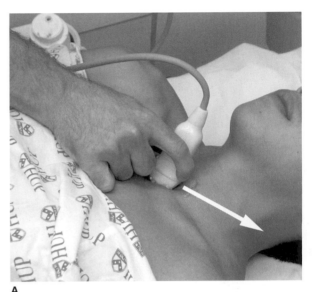

A

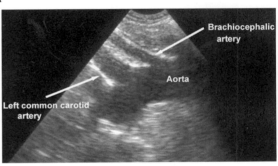

B

Figure 8.10 Suprasternal views of the aortic arch. **(A)** Probe positioning for suprasternal views of the aortic arch. The arrow indicates the direction of the probe "pointer" approximately 30 degrees clockwise from the sagittal plane. Ideally, a small footprint probe should be utilised, and, if tolerated by the patient, a bolster should be placed under the shoulders to maximally extend the neck. **(B)** Suprasternal view of the ascending aorta. The aortic root is on the right of the image, the arch (obscured in this image) would be on the left.

the arch (see Figures 8.10A and 8.10B). Distal dissection is not usually a cause of shock _per se_, however, if distal dissection is identified it may provide the necessary confirmation of an extended proximal dissection which escaped detection on transthoracic evaluation. For this reason, in the appropriate clinical setting, the abdominal aorta can also be evaluated for evidence of dissection (see Case 4 and Figure 8.4B). Even without an identifiable intimal flap, a patient with symptoms of dissection, hypotension, and pericardial effusion should prompt consideration of cardiac tamponade, which is the single most deadly complication of aortic dissection.

Pleural and pulmonary abnormalities

Although the physical findings of tension pneumothorax are familiar to the emergency physician, they can be overlooked in the frenetic activity of diagnosing and resuscitating a hypotensive patient. The use of ultrasound in the diagnosis of pneumothorax is well described.[22–24] In the supine patient, the probe (ideally a 6–12 MHz linear array) is placed perpendicular to the ribs in the second to fourth intercostal spaces in the midclavicular line. The ribs have superficially echogenic surfaces, which cast intense acoustical shadows. Between the ribs, and usually 3–5 mm deeper, the brightly echogenic line of the pleura can be identified. Under normal circumstances, respirophasic "lung sliding" caused by the movement of the lung and visceral pleura adjacent to the parietal pleura can be seen. The identification of pleural sliding may be facilitated by the use of power Doppler, if available. Pneumothorax is diagnosed by the absence of this (see Chapter 5).

Another finding, mobile, transient, comet tail artefacts arising from the pleural line, also rules out pneumothorax (see Figure 8.11). These narrow comet tail artefacts are thought to arise from air filled bronchioles embedded in oedematous lung tissue immediately below the visceral pleura. Occasional comet tail artefacts may be of no clinical significance, but when seen copiously, they are a sign of "wet lung" (increased interstitial pulmonary fluid), the many causes of which include congestive heart failure, sepsis, trauma, and aspiration. These must be distinguished from the wide linear reverberation artefacts seen in both normal lung and pneumothorax, which extend below the pleura at a distance approximately equal to that between the probe surface and the pleura. Another finding inconstantly identified in pneumothorax is the "lung-point sign", caused by the movement under the transducer, of the line of demarcation between collapsed and uncollapsed lung. In the context of a hypotensive patient, additional findings which might suggest the presence of tension pneumothorax include difficulty locating the heart and/or marked lateral displacement of the usual cardiac windows. False positive results for absence of lung sliding may arise due to pleural scarring, pleurodesis, large pulmonic blebs, or the noncompliant lungs of adult respiratory distress syndrome. Conversely, with a normal sonographic evaluation despite a clinical picture

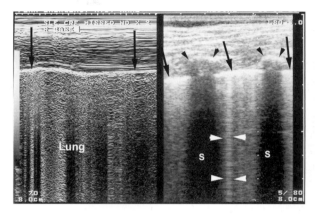

Figure 8.11 Ultrasound findings in "wet lung". The right hand side of the figure is a B-Mode image showing ribs (black arrowheads), which can be recognised by their intense shadows (S). The bright echogenic line of the pleura (black arrows) lies immediately below the ribs. In real-time this is examined for pleural sliding. In this patient in renal failure and volume overload, the pleural line gave rise to numerous comet tail artefacts (white arrowheads), indicative of "wet lung". The left hand side of the image is a simultaneous M-Mode record. The pleural line is again easily identifiable (black arrows), and the granular quality generated by subpleural lung rules out pneumothorax.

strongly suggestive of pneumothorax, other intercostal windows should be evaluated, especially those with diminished breath sounds.

Occasionally a massive pleural effusion will be responsible for hypotension, often associated with respiratory compromise. A variety of sonographic findings have been described. The two of most relevance in the hypotensive patient are the characteristic layering, echogenic appearance of empyema; and the identification of a net-like web of septations indicating loculated effusion, which will resist efforts of drainage by means of pleurocentesis (see Figure 13.14).[25] Another finding which may be encountered in an EMBU evaluation of the thorax in a critically ill, septic patient is massive pulmonary consolidation. The ultrasound examination is remarkable for lung tissue which is sonolucent with irregular patchy disorganised internal echoes often with foci of ring down artefact caused by air-filled bronchi, which retains typical pulmonary respirophasic motion. Other sonographic characteristics of lung consolidation which distinguish it from other lesions of the lung or pleura include a wedge shape, being well defined peripherally by pleura, but poorly defined centrally, and the presence of air and fluid bronchograms (see Figure 8.12).[26]

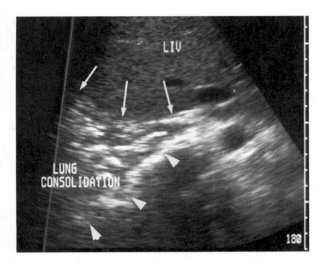

Figure 8.12 Lung consolidation in pneumonia. In this right upper quadrant view using the liver as a window, the usual mirror artefact at the diaphragm (arrows) is lost, and a wedge shaped area of lung consolidation, defined peripherally by the pleura, with poor central definition is clearly seen. It has irregular internal echodensities, and unlike normal tissue transmits ultrasound effectively, providing a clear image of the costal pleura (arrowheads).

Evaluation of the abdomen and pneumoperitoneum

The sonographic features of abdominal aortic aneurysm are considered in detail elsewhere in this text. Tension pneumoperitoneum is rare, so that pneumoperitoneum is not usually a cause of hypotension *per se;* however, elderly patients with hypotension due to sepsis arising from a perforated abdominal viscus often present with obtundation that precludes effective clinical assessment. In the diagnosis of pneumoperitoneum, sonography has been shown to be more reliable than the plain film radiographs on which emergency physicians have traditionally relied. The technique is similar to that used in the identification of pneumothorax: in the normal state, the parietal peritoneum can be identified as a thin, bright, echogenic line below the muscle layers and preperitoneal fat of the abdominal wall. Beneath this echogenic line on the ultrasound screen, the abdominal contents can be seen sliding back and forth with respirations. Peristalsis may also be noted.

With pneumoperitoneum, in addition to the absence of these findings, the line of the parietal peritoneum becomes intensely echogenic. A large pneumoperitoneum is often signalled by unexpected difficulty in obtaining any images of abdominal contents, which the inexperienced sonologist may ascribe to "bowel gas". This finding is analogous to that of tension pneumothorax, which, as noted above, may reveal itself to the physician by causing extraordinary and inexplicable difficulty in obtaining adequate views of the heart. Smaller volumes of free air give rise to focal areas of intense echoing at the level of the parietal peritoneum with intense reverberation artefact extending downwards on the ultrasound screen. If pneumoperitoneum is not obvious, careful examination of both the epigastrium and right hypochondrium in both supine and left side down lateral decubitus positions should be performed. Occasionally air-filled bowel immediately below the peritoneum can cause confusion, although intraluminal gas, with its characteristic "corrugated" pattern caused by its location between the folds of the bowel wall, its physically contained and delimited extent, and its peristalsis, usually distinguishes it from free air. In situations of doubt, the patient should be placed in a left decubitus position, since free air shifts much more extensively and freely than loops of gas-filled bowel.

Sonography in the evaluation of shortness of breath and/or dyspnoea

Most causes of dyspnoea are either pulmonary or cardiac; and these can usually be distinguished on clinical grounds. However, non-cardiac circulatory embarrassment can also cause respiratory complaints, as seen in Cases 1 and 2; and in some frequently encountered ED populations, such as elderly patients with a history of both chronic lung disease and atherosclerotic cardiovascular disease, the distinction may not be clear. In addition, pulmonary embolus and pericardial effusion/tamponade mandate specific therapeutic interventions and are not easily identifiable with the basic tests immediately available in most EDs: blood work, ECG, and chest radiographs. Causes of dyspnoea identifiable by EMBU are listed in the following box. The sonographic findings associated with these were considered above in the discussion of unexplained hypotension.

Causes of shortness of breath or dyspnoea identifiable with sonography
EMBU of the chest
Pericardial effusion and/or tamponade
Pulmonary embolus
Massive pleural effusion
Pneumothorax or tension pneumothorax
"Wet lung": congestive heart failure, volume overload, adult respiratory distress syndrome, etc
Lower extremity compression sonography
Deep vein thrombosis

Causes of pulseless electrical activity
Mechanical causes potentially amenable to therapeutic intervention
Pericardial tamponade*
Pulmonary embolus #
Intravascular volume depletion and/or massive intracavitary haemorrhage*
Tension pneumothorax #
Acute myocardial infarction #
Non-mechanical causes potentially amenable to therapeutic intervention
Electrolyte abnormalities, especially hyperkalaemia
Acid base disturbances, especially acidosis
Hypoxia
Hypothermia
Toxins
Coronary ischaemia
"Irreversible" causes
Any of the above leading to massive and irreversible myocardial injury
*Indicates causes that can be ruled out by EMBU #Indicates causes that can be ruled in, but not excluded by EMBU

One study in which EMBU of the heart and lower extremities was used in the initial evaluation of patients with undifferentiated dyspnoea, found that 31% had sonographic findings which altered the diagnostic evaluation.[27] The most commonly identified abnormality was depressed left ventricular function. In another study, cardiac EMBU was performed on patients whose dyspnoea was unexplained after a full work-up, which included (as clinically indicated) blood tests, ECG, chest radiographs, and ventilation-perfusion scanning. A total of 14% of these patients were found to have pericardial effusions; 4% with large effusions requiring pericardiocentesis, 3% with moderate effusions requiring admission and observation.[28]

Sonography in the evaluation of pulseless electrical activity and cardiopulmonary arrest

Cardiopulmonary arrest is the final common pathway of progressive respiratory and circulatory insufficiency. Several uses of EMBU as an adjunct to cardiopulmonary resuscitation (CPR) have been described. It can provide diagnoses, assistance in the performance of invasive procedures, information as to their efficacy, and guidance in termination of resuscitation efforts. Many such studies have used transoesophageal echocardiography (TEE). The findings of these studies are relevant, despite the fact that many EDs do not yet possess TEE, for two reasons. First, while TEE affords a more complete and detailed view of the heart, ascending, and descending aorta, and has been shown to be a more accurate diagnostic test, transthoracic echocardiography (TTE) can still provide valuable information in situations where

the former is not available. Second, TTE, a non-invasive test, will always be capable of more rapid deployment without the risks of aspiration and sedation associated with TEE. Both of these reasons are borne out in Case 4. Third, with increasing familiarity with ultrasound, it is likely that the availability and use of TEE will become more widespread.

Pulseless electrical activity (PEA) is defined as "electrical activity that can be seen on the monitor … although the patient lacks a detectable pulse".[29] Causes of PEA are traditionally separated into those that are potentially reversible, and those that are not (see box above). Reversible causes can be further subdivided into those that are mechanical (pulmonary embolism, pericardial tamponade, hypovolaemia, tension pneumothorax) and those that are metabolic (hyperkalaemia, acidosis, drug overdose). Irreversible causes are usually related to global myocardial dysfunction, either from prolonged insult from a reversible cause, or due to massive myocardial infarction.[30]

Sonography has shown that the majority of patients in PEA have some myocardial activity, and that a spectrum of cardiac activity may occur with apparent pulselessness in PEA. This spectrum reflects a continuum of progressively increasing myocardial compromise.

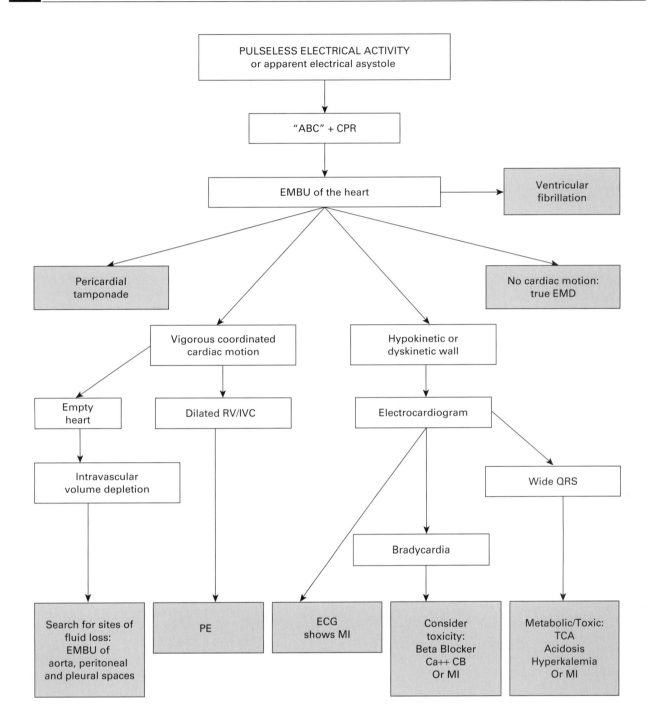

Figure 8.13 Possible algorithm for use of EMBU in the management of pulseless electrical activity. (Tinted boxes are end-points with specific management or therapy.)

- The heart is intrinsically healthy, but circulatory failure occurs due to a mechanical derangement (for example hypovolaemia or pulmonary embolus).
- A moderately damaged myocardium makes concerted but weak contractions generating low, non-palpable blood pressures.
- A severely injured myocardium contracts in time with its electrical activity, but so weakly that valve closure is not achieved.
- The myocardium has absolutely no activity. This state has been referred to as "true electromechanical dissociation".

In addition to this continuum, so-called "pseudo PEA" has been described in which an adequately pumping heart fails to generate pulses due to severe vasoconstriction.

The first group of patients in the spectrum of PEA are those with intrinsically healthy hearts with a non-cardiac cause for circulatory arrest. Most of these patients are in the group with reversible mechanical causes of PEA. Treatment of these diseases depends on rapid and specific interventions; this, in turn, depends on timely diagnosis. Most mechanical causes of PEA are identifiable by ultrasound, as noted in the box above. Diagnostic accuracy is essential since their management is, in many cases, mutually exclusive. For example, massive pulmonary embolus is treated with anticoagulation and thrombolysis, both of which are contraindicated in cardiac tamponade. The proportion of patients with PEA or cardiopulmonary arrest whose cause is reversible is not known, but studies have shown a range from 20–35%.[31,32] For this reason, the American Heart Association currently advocates echocardiography as a component of the "Primary ABC … Survey" of PEA.[29]

An algorithm for the use of EMBU in the management of patients in PEA or apparent electrical asystole is shown in Figure 8.13. PEA is initially diagnosed by physical examination and cardiac monitor. As suggested by this flow chart, many of the reversible causes of PEA are immediately identifiable by EMBU, and are not further elucidated by ECG, so this should be the first step after initiation of supportive measures. EMBU will immediately diagnose complete absence of cardiac activity (true electromechanical dissociation), and pericardial tamponade. Patients are then divided by the sonographic findings into those with, and those without, coordinated vigorous cardiac activity. In those with vigorous myocardial contractility, patients with intravascular volume depletion can be distinguished from those with acute massive PE, as noted in the discussion of unexplained hypotension. Diffusely hypokinetic contractions are likely to be due to massive MI and/or severe metabolic/toxic derangements. These may be elucidated with a 12-lead ECG. Focal areas of hypokinesis or dyskinesis are likely to be due to acute ischaemic insult, although, as noted above, isolated right ventricular dysfunction and dilation may be due to massive PE as well as RV infarct.

While cardiopulmonary arrest takes many forms in addition to PEA, the two have many causes in common, as shown in studies that use sonography in the setting of CPR.[32,33] In addition to identifying mechanical causes, in a manner analogous to that for PEA, sonography has been used to diagnose ventricular fibrillation during apparent asystole by ECG monitoring[33,34]; and to identify pacemaker placement and capture during CPR.[33,35–37] With the exceedingly small proportion of patients who survive CPA to hospital discharge, sonography can also help guide decisions about termination of resuscitation. While studies have found that complete cardiac standstill is an almost universal predictor of unsuccessful resuscitation, exceptions have been observed[37]; although the latter study only recorded ED survival to hospital admission. Even in the absence of an immutable rule, it is likely that identification of cardiac standstill would be the most definitive way of showing that the patient had met the ACLS recommended criteria for termination of CPR: asystole despite implementation of applicable ACLS protocols. Another finding that may be seen in unsuccessful resuscitation is diffuse "gel-like" echodensities filling the cardiac chambers: presumably coagulating blood. This has been described in the literature, but never studied prospectively as a marker of death.[31,33]

Summary

EMBU has been developed for the evaluation of critically ill emergency patients. Although technically more challenging and complex, the case scenarios illustrate that emergency ultrasound can be used to assess medical causes of unexplained hypotension and shortness of breath, affording rapid diagnosis and allowing early treatment. An integrated approach of clinical assessment and EMBU will lead to improved care of critically ill patients.

References

1 Rozycki GS, Shackford SR. Ultrasound, what every surgeon should know. *J Trauma* 1996;**40(1)**:1–4.

2 American Medical Association House of Delegates Resolution 802, 1999.

3 Rose JS, Bair AE, Mandavia D, Kinser DJ. The UHP ultrasound protocol: a novel ultrasound approach to the empiric evaluation of the undifferentiated hypotensive patient. *Am J Emerg Med* 2001;**19(4)**:299–302.

4 Hendrickson RG, Dean AJ, Costantino TG. A novel use of ultrasound in pulseless electrical activity: the diagnosis of an acute abdominal aortic aneurysm rupture. *J Emerg Med* 2001;**21(2)**:141–4.

5 Kimura BJ, Pezeshki B, Frack SA, DeMaria AN. Feasibility of "limited" echo imaging: characterization of incidental findings. *J Am Soc Echocardiogr* 1998;**11(7)**:746–50.

6 Kimura BJ, Amundson SA, Willis CL, Gilpin EA, DeMaria AN. Usefulness of a hand-held ultrasound device for bedside examination of left ventricular function. *Am J Cardiol* 2002;**90(9)**:1038–9.

7 Rugolotto M, Chang CP, Hu B, Schnittger I, Liang DH. Clinical use of cardiac ultrasound performed with a hand-carried device in patients admitted for acute cardiac care. *Am J Cardiol* 2002;**90(9)**:1040–2.

8 Moore CL, Rose GA, Tayal VS, Sullivan M, Arrowood JA, Kline JA. Determination of left ventricular function by emergency physician echocardiography of hypotensive patients. *Acad Emerg Med* 2002;**9**:189–93.

9 Lipton B. Estimation of central venous pressure by ultrasound of the internal jugular vein. *Am J Emerg Med* 2000;**18**:432–4.

10 Oh JK, Miller FA, Shub C, Reeder GS, Tajik AJ. Evaluation of acute chest pain syndromes by two-dimensional echocardiography: its potential application in the selection of patients for acute reperfusion therapy. *Mayo Clinic Proc* 1987;**62(1)**:59–66.

11 Stamm RB, Carabello BA, Mayers DL, Martin RP. Two-dimensional echocardiographic measurement of left ventricular ejection fraction: prospective analysis of what constitutes an adequate determination. *Am Heart J* 1982;**104(1)**:136–44.

12 Mueller X, Stauffer JC, Jaussi A, Goy JJ, Kappenberger L. Subjective visual echocardiographic estimate of left ventricular ejection fraction as an alternative to conventional echocardiographic methods: comparison with contrast angiography. *Clin Cardiol* 1991;**14(11)**:898–902.

13 Amico AF, Lichtenberg GS, Reisner SA, Stone CK, Schwartz RG, Meltzer RS. Superiority of visual versus computerized echocardiographic estimation of radionuclide left ventricular ejection fraction. *Am Heart J* 1989;**118(6)**:1259–65.

14 Jackson RE, Rudoni RR, Hauser AM, Pascual RG, Hussey ME. Prospective evaluation of two-dimensional transthoracic echocardiography in emergency department patients with suspected pulmonary embolism. *Acad Emerg Med* 2000;**7(9)**:994–8.

15 Grifoni S, Olivotto I, Cecchini P, *et al.* Utility of an integrated clinical, echocardiographic, and venous ultrasonographic approach for triage of patients with suspected pulmonary embolism. *Am J Cardiol* 1998;**82(10)**:1230–5.

16 Rudoni RR, Jackson RE, Godfrey GW, Bonfiglio AX, Hussey ME, Hauser AM. Use of two-dimensional echocardiography in the diagnosis of pulmonary embolus. *J Emerg Med* 1998;**6(1)**:5–8.

17 Weston MJ, Wilde P. Echocardiographic diagnosis of massive pulmonary embolism. *Br J Radiol* 1989;**2(740)**:751–3.

18 Wellford AL, Snoey ER. Emergency medicine applications of echocardiography. *Emerg Med Clin North Am* 1995;**13(4)**:831–54.

19 Cheriex EC, Sreeram N, Eussen YFJM, Pieters FAA, Wellens HJJ. Cross sectional Doppler echocardiography as the initial technique for the diagnosis of acute pulmonary embolism. *Br Heart J* 1994;**72**:52–7.

20 Kinch JW, Ryan TJ. Right ventricular infarction. *N Engl J Med* 1994;**330(17)**:1211–7.

21 Steiner P, Lund GK, Debatin JF, *et al.* Acute pulmonary embolism: value of transthoracic and transesophageal echocardiography in comparison with helical CT. *Am J Dent* 1996;**167**:931–6.

22 Wernecke K, Galanski M, Peters PE, Hansen J. Pneumothorax: evaluation by ultrasound – preliminary results. *J Thor Imag* 1987;**2(2)**:76–8.

23 Dulchavsky SA, Schwarz KL, Kirkpatrick AW, *et al.* Prospective evaluation of thoracic ultrasound in the detection of pneumothorax. *J Trauma* 2001;**50(2)**:201–5.

24 Chan SSW. Emergency bedside ultrasound to detect pneumothorax. *Acad Emerg Med* 2003;**10(1)**:91–4.

25 Gryminski J, Pawlicka L. Ultrasound pattern of pleural effusions of various origin: a study based on 1000 patients with pleural effusion. *Chest* 1997;**112(3)**Supp 3:12S.

26 Brant WE. Chest. In McGahan JP, Goldberg BB, eds. *Diagnostic Ultrasound: a logical approach.* Philadelphia: Lippincott-Raven, 1998;1063–81.

27 Dawson BJ, Moore CL, Lambert MJ. EPISODE: emergency physician impact of sonography on dyspnea evaluation. *Ann Emerg Med* 2002;**40(4)**:S74.

28 Blaivas M. Incidence of pericardial effusion in patients presenting to the emergency department

with unexplained dyspnea. *Acad Emerg Med* 2001;**8(12)**:1143–6.

29 Cummins RO, ed. *ACLS Provider Manual.* American Heart Association, 2001, p107.

30 Committee on Emergency Cardiac Care and Subcommittee on Advanced Cardiac Life Support. *Textbook of Advanced Cardiac Life Support.* American Heart Association, 1994.

31 Varriale P, Maldonado JM. Echocardiographic observations during inhospital cardiopulmonary resuscitation. *Crit Care Med* 1997;**25(10)**:1717–20.

32 van der Wouw PA, Koster RW, Dellemarre BJ, *et al.* Diagnostic accuracy of transesophageal echocardiography during cardiopulmonary resuscitation. *J Am Coll Cardiol* 1997;**30(3)**:780–3.

33 Wright RF. Clinical utility of transesophageal echocardiography during cardiopulmonary resuscitation. *Circulation* 1995;**88**:190–2.

34 Amaya SC, Langsam A. Ultrasound detection of ventricular fibrillation disguised as asystole. *Ann Emerg Med* 1999;**33**:344–6.

35 Macedo W Jr, Sturmann K, Kim JM, Kang J. Ultrasonographic guidance of transvenous pacemaker insertion in the emergency department: a report of three cases. *J Emerg Med* 1999;**17(3)**: 491–6.

36 Aguilera PA, Durham BA, Riley DA. Emergency transvenous cardiac pacing placement using ultrasound guidance. *Ann Emerg Med* 2000;**36(3)**: 224–7.

37 Salen P, O'Connor R, Sierzenski P, *et al.* Can cardiac sonography and capnography be used independently and in combination to predict resuscitation outcomes? *Acad Emerg Med* 2001; **8(6)**:610–5.

9 Obstetric and gynaecological emergencies

ANDREW LOUGHNEY, STEPHEN STIRGESS

Objectives
To review the role of ultrasound in:
- gynaecological emergencies
- early pregnancy
- the second and third trimester of pregnancy
- labour

Introduction

The Confidential Enquiries into Maternal Deaths (*Why Mothers Die*) is a review document published once every three years, detailing each pregnancy-related maternal death in the United Kingdom. In its latest edition, the report illustrated that a woman giving birth in an emergency department was proportionately more likely to die during the process than a woman giving birth in any other setting. This reflects the fact that women frequently attend emergency departments rather than seeking obstetric, gynaecological, or midwifery care when experiencing what they regard as urgent medical problems, whatever the nature of the symptoms. It is important therefore that emergency physicians retain a good working knowledge of acute obstetric and gynaecological illnesses and are proficient in the initial management of cases.

Ultrasound is central to the modern practice of obstetrics and gynaecology, playing a role both in diagnosis and in the execution of practical procedures. This has been true in the non-acute arena for a considerable time, but more recently the use of ultrasound in acute areas of practice has gained greater prominence. For example, the authors of a discussion document produced by the Royal College of Obstetricians and Gynaecologists entitled *Towards Safer Childbirth* suggested that portable ultrasound facilities should be available on every consultant led delivery suite and that staff should be trained to be proficient in its use. As a result, the scope of ultrasound in facilitating the safe provision of intrapartum care has expanded rapidly,[1] as it has in other areas of acute obstetric and gynaecological practice. In the following chapter, we will discuss the role of ultrasound in the management of emergencies in three areas:

- gynaecology, including early pregnancy
- second and third trimester of pregnancy
- intrapartum care.

The practical application of ultrasound in the assessment of the woman and, where applicable, the fetus will form the focus of this text. Realistically achievable targets will be delineated for practitioners in emergency medicine.

Gynaecology

The gynaecological symptoms most likely to bring a woman to an emergency department are pelvic pain, abnormal vaginal bleeding, or a combination of both. In general, initial diagnosis and management will rest upon the results of two investigations:

- pregnancy testing
- trans vaginal (TV) ultrasound.

The principles involved in performing these tests will be presented in the following section. Acute problems associated with early pregnancy, ovarian accidents, and pelvic inflammatory disease will then be explored since these are the gynaecological conditions most commonly encountered in the emergency department.

Pregnancy testing

Ultrasound needs to be interpreted alongside other investigations, specifically pregnancy testing. A developing conceptus releases human chorion gonadotrophin (hCG) into the maternal circulation, the β subunit of which may be detected in a non-quantitative urinary bedside kit as little as two weeks after conception. The test is simple to perform and has a negligible false positive rate. Furthermore, 'false' negative results will only occur in the very earliest stages of pregnancy or more than two weeks after fetoplacental demise, when clinically significant pregnancy related diseases are improbable. Since the result of a pregnancy test run from a midstream or catheterised sample of urine takes little over a minute to obtain, the test is invaluable in determining whether acute gynaecological presentations are related to early pregnancy or not.

Serum assays for β hCG are also available in most hospitals as a laboratory test. They hold the advantage that they are quantitative and this can be useful in the management of early pregnancy problems.

Trans vaginal scanning

When trying to determine the nature of a gynaecological disease, TV scanning is essential because the vaginal probe sits close to the uterus and can be angled easily towards the pelvic adnexae. This aids tissue penetration and allows the operator to use a relatively high (5·0–7·5 MHz) transducer frequency, thereby improving picture resolution. As a result, TV scanning is more sensitive to the presence of small but clinically significant pelvic structures than abdominal scanning.

Patient

The patient first empties her bladder then, in a suitably private environment, she adopts a supine position with her sacrum adjacent to the end of an examination couch.

Her feet rest at the height of a chair seat (Figure 9.1).

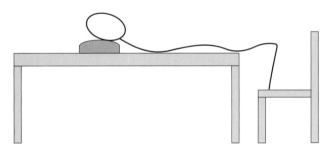

Figure 9.1 Supine woman on examination couch.

Probe position

Cover with disposable condom and apply gel to outside.

Insert gently into lower third of vagina, insonated in sagittal plane.

Angle tip of probe downwards and posteriorly. Swing probe anteriorly to view whole of uterus in longtitudinal axis from fundus to cervix (Figure 9.2).

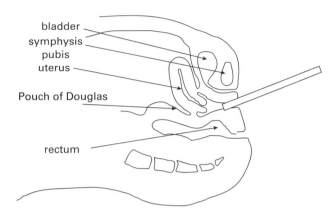

Figure 9.2 Vaginal probe in female pelvis.

Minor adjustments allow examination of the remaining uterine contour from the right side to the left and from the anterior to the posterior wall. The appearance of the cervix and cervical canal are noted at this point and the thickness of endometrium measured in the sagittal plane. The probe is then swung further anteriorly to reveal the bladder and its contents, then posteriorly to reveal the contents of the Pouch of Douglas.

To view the adnexae, the probe is rotated 90 degrees clockwise into the coronal plane and the tip tilted towards the right side of the pelvis. This allows identification of the right internal iliac artery and vein (Figure 9.3). The ovary is most commonly found anterior and medial to these vessels, although its position may vary. The tip of the probe is then swept into the midline without additional rotation, to allow examination of the uterus and its cavity in the coronal plane. Finally, the probe is angled towards the left side of the pelvis, again without rotation. This allows identification of the left internal iliac vessels and the left ovary, together with any structures such as cysts, abscesses, or a gestational sac occuring in association with the adnexal tissues.

The first trimester of pregnancy

Although nausea, vomiting, and general malaise are common in the first trimester, the two symptoms most likely to bring a woman to an emergency department are:

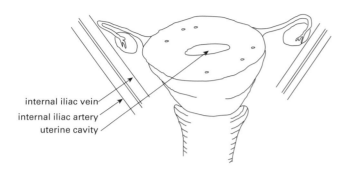

internal iliac vein
internal iliac artery
uterine cavity

Figure 9.3   Female pelvis with lateral structures.

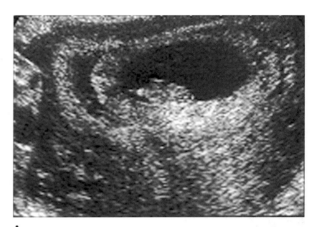

A

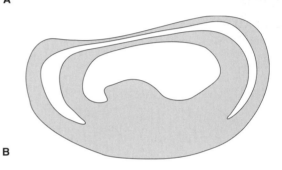

B

Figure 9.4   The double ring in early pregnancy. The initial formation of fetal tissue can be seen.

* pain
* vaginal bleeding.

The initial management of a woman presenting with pain or bleeding in early pregnancy should be determined by her haemodynamic status. Both ectopic pregnancy and miscarriage can be associated with massive haemorrhage and this may be concealed in nature. Therefore basic resuscitative measures including adequate fluid replacement therapy should be instituted before any attempt is made to refine a diagnosis.

The distinction must then be made between the threatened or inevitable miscarriage of an intrauterine pregnancy and ectopic pregnancy. The presenting history is often helpful in this respect since threatened miscarriage is commonly associated with moderate vaginal blood loss shortly followed by suprapubic pain and low, central backache. The pain associated with an ectopic pregnancy in contrast tends to precede vaginal bleeding and to be more severe in nature. These clinical distinctions are however unreliable. A pregnancy implanted in a fallopian tube may be painless until it ruptures for example, and vaginal bleeding is not always apparent even after rupture. As a result in most cases, the diagnosis rests with ultrasound.

When the conceptus has implanted and is developing within the uterine cavity, a gestational sac may be seen on TV scanning four to five weeks after the start of the last menstrual period. To confirm the presence of an intrauterine pregnancy at this stage, the sonographic appearance of a double ring must be identified, the inner ring representing the chorionic sac and

Table 9.1

Crown Rump Length (mm)	Gestation (weeks)
4·5	6
10	7
16	8
23	9
31	10
41	11
52	12

the outer ring representing decidualised endometrium (Figure 9.4A and B).

Intrauterine fetal parts are first discernible during the fifth week and after this time, measurement of the length of the fetus from crown to rump will give an estimate of gestational age (Figure 9.5A and B and Table 9.1). Further sonographic landmarks include the identification of a fetal heart beat by the end of the fifth week and

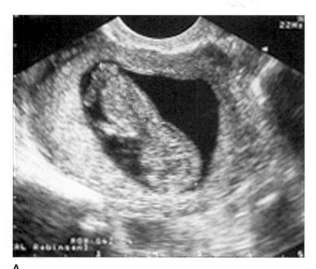

A

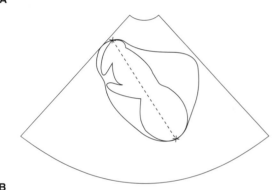

B

Figure 9.5 Fetus showing crown rump length. Fetal movement and the presence of a heart beat confirmed viability despite bleeding per vaginam.

the presence of fetal movements by the end of the seventh. These signs indicate that the pregnancy is ongoing even in the presence of bleeding and pain.

When a fetus fails to meet these landmarks, miscarriage is likely but immediate medical or surgical uterine evacuation should only be contemplated if the patient is haemodynamically unstable. A second TV scan will usually be required one week later to confirm the diagnosis since this will exclude errors that may be made in calculating the gestational age of the pregnancy. Falling serum levels of β hCG will also be found when a pregnancy is miscarrying, whereas rising levels will accompany ongoing pregnancy.

A pregnancy ectopically implanted into a fallopian tube, ovary, or other distant site may also be associated with the accumulation of fluid in the uterine lumen at five weeks' gestation. The absence of a chorionic sac however leads to the appearance of only a single ring or "pseudosac" in

the uterus, in contrast to the double ring of an intrauterine pregnancy. The identification of a cystic mass with complex shadows in the adnexa may give a further clue to the presence of an ectopic pregnancy, although it is often impossible to determine the exact site of origin of such a mass on ultrasound. Finally, bleeding associated with ectopic pregnancy may manifest itself as free fluid in the Pouch of Douglas.

> **Pitfalls**
>
> Ectopic pregnancy can occur in the absence of either a single uterine ring, an adnexal mass, or free peritoneal fluid.
>
> Diagnosis will then rest on the presence of a positive pregnancy test, with a serum β hCG over 1000 iu/ml and an empty uterus on TV scanning.
>
> These features should trigger urgent liaison with a gynaecologist, and may lead to laparoscopy for confirmation of the diagnosis and treatment of the condition.

Ovarian accidents   Mild to moderate pelvic pain commonly arises in conjunction with menstrual disorders. When pain is severe enough to bring a non-pregnant woman to an emergency department however, it is more likely to be caused either by an accident (rupture or torsion) involving an ovarian cyst or by acute pelvic inflammatory disease (PID). In each case, signs of peritonitis may be elicited on abdominal examination and digital pelvic examination is likely to be painful. The presence of tachycardia, low grade pyrexia, and a modest leucocytosis is also common to each of these conditions. TV scanning can however be used to differentiate between them.

The sonographic appearances of ovarian cysts vary with their pathological origin. For all ovarian lesions however, the presence of septa, the number of loculi present, and the presence of solid areas within the cyst should always be noted when a TV scan is performed. The diameter of the ovary should also be measured in a parasagittal (D1), anteroposterior (D2), and transverse (D3) plane (Figure 9.6) so that its approximate volume can be calculated:

$$\text{Volume} = 0.52 \times D1 \times D2 \times D3$$

The appearance of fluid in the Pouch of Douglas suggests rupture of a cyst and possible associated haemorrhage. Although this may cause considerable pain, the blood loss is rarely sufficient to compromise the patient's circulatory state. Liaison with gynaecological services would be appropriate in most cases rather than looking for immediate operative intervention.

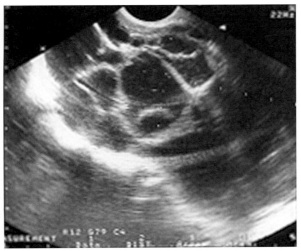

A

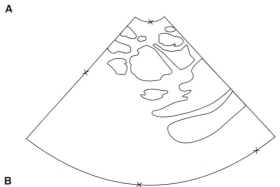

B

Figure 9.6 A large ovarian cyst.

Pitfalls

A small amount of fluid may also be seen in the Pouch of Douglas in association with torsion of an ovarian cyst, this representing transudate rather than blood.

Torsion usually also involves the ipsilateral fallopian tube.

As a result the tube can often be seen as a tortuous, distended, cystic structure in the adnexa with thickened walls and incomplete septa.

It is not always possible to distinguish the tube from the ovary on ultrasound in these circumstances and the final diagnosis may then not be made until laparoscopy is carried out.

Pelvic inflammatory disease

Pelvic inflammatory disease (PID) arises when sexually transmitted organisms infect the tissues lining the uterine cavity, fallopian tubes, adnexal tissues, or the pelvic visceral peritoneum. Since acute salpingitis is associated with severe lower abdominal pain, this condition is frequently encountered in the emergency department. Rapid diagnosis and treatment is important because

without this, infertility will arise in up to 20% of women while approximately 3% will later experience an ectopic pregnancy. To this end, TV ultrasound may be used to detect small abscesses in the uterine cavity, fallopian tube, ovary, or peritoneum. Thickening and distortion of the fallopian tube may also be detected.[2]

Pitfalls

Absence of these ultrasonographic features does not exclude the diagnosis of PID.

As a result, whenever the clinician suspects PID, microbiological pelvic swabs should be taken in addition to an endocervical chlamydial swab.

Treatment with broad spectrum antibiotics should be instituted before obtaining formal bacteriological culture results when the index of suspicion is high.

Second and third trimester of pregnancy

Second trimester abdominal ultrasound scans have established an important role in obstetric practice, particularly in identifying fetal structural abnormalities. The emergency physician is more likely to use ultrasound in the second and third trimester however when a woman presents with an acute medical problem such as:

- pain
- bleeding
- reduced fetal movements
- prelabour rupture of the membranes.

In this section the technique of abdominal scanning during the second and third trimesters of pregnancy is described. Identification of the fetal heart beat, fetal activity, measurement of liquor volume, and placental characterisation will then be discussed using a combination of abdominal and TV scanning, since the ability to carry out these investigations will enable the emergency physician to manage acute clinical presentations safely.

Abdominal scanning

Patient

The patient does not need to have a full bladder before an obstetric abdominal ultrasound scan is commenced, but this may be advantageous if the cervix and adjacent structures are to be visualised. Hydration with oral or intravenous fluid will achieve this within 30 minutes, but infusion of the bladder with 500 ml saline via a catheter is more rapid and will have the same effect.

The patient adopts a supine position on an examination couch. Approximately 15 degrees of left lateral pelvic tilt will relieve vena caval obstruction and facilitate venous return from the lower limbs, minimising the risk of postural hypotension. This can be obtained by placing the edge of a pillow under the patient's right buttock if the examination couch does not have a tilt facility.

The abdomen is then exposed from xiphisternum to symphysis pubis and ultrasound gel applied to the skin above the symphysis.

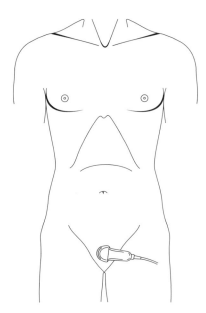

Figure 9.7 Positioning of abdominal probe.

Probe

A 3·5–5 MHz abdominal transducer is applied perpendicularly to the skin to give a midline sagittal view of the lower half of the uterus. The caudal structures are seen uppermost on the monitor (Figure 9.7).

Parasagittal views are obtained by moving the transducer towards the left and the right iliac fossae while maintaining its perpendicular plane.

The contents of the upper portion of the uterus can be seen by angling the probe towards the uterine fundus, but simply repositioning the transducer above the umbilicus will also achieve this while helping the operator to maintain orientation.

When specific structures are being examined in detail, the probe may be rotated up to 90 degrees clockwise or anticlockwise to obtain the desired view. Structures to the left or right hand side of the maternal abdomen respectively will then appear uppermost on the monitor.

Fetal assessment

The most basic measure of fetal well being in pregnancy lies with the identification of a fetal heart beat (FH). Hand held Doppler devices can generally be used for this purpose but if the FH cannot be identified with this simple approach, abdominal ultrasound should be used to determine whether or not the fetus is alive. To do this, a clear, four-chamber view of the heart should be obtained by positioning the transducer to give a transverse view through the fetal chest (Figure 9.8A and B). Although the cardiac outline will usually be clearly delineated in this way, the tissues are less well defined if fetal death has occurred several days prior to presentation at the hospital.

Pitfalls

Asystole should only be confirmed by an experienced operator, after continuous scanning for several minutes to exclude profound, prolonged bradycardia.

The presence of an FH does not in itself exclude the presence of chronic or acute fetal hypoxia. A Doppler based cardiotocographic trace (CTG) may be used to add a level of sophistication to the assessment of the FH, since variation in some of the CTG's features can point to the presence of fetal hypoxia. In addition however, it is known that a healthy fetus exhibits quiet and active behavioural states alternately over time. In the active state, gross fetal body movements and fetal breathing movements may be seen on ultrasound scanning. Loss of these coordinated movements accompanies chronic hypoxia when this is severe enough to affect the central nervous system. This phenomenon may be identified by abdominal ultrasound, although observation for at least 40 minutes is required before a significant change in behaviour can be recorded reliably. Such changes in the fetal behavioural state are particularly useful in assessing the well being of a fetus in utero when concern arises because of a reported lack of fetal movements felt by the pregnant woman.

Liquor

Beyond 20 weeks, gestation, most of the liquor bathing the fetus is produced by the passage of urine. To achieve a balanced volume in the amniotic sac, the fetus ingests liquor and any

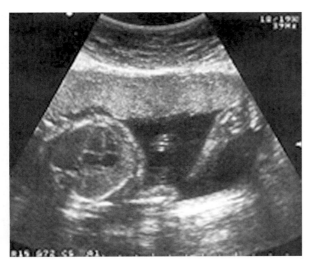

A

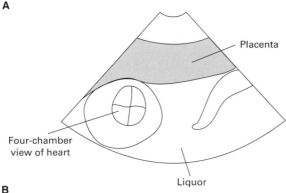

B

Figure 9.8 Four-chamber view of the fetal heart. Placental tissue can be seen anterially, liquor laterally.

excess fluid is removed via the placenta. A fall in liquor volume (oligohydramnios) most commonly accompanies loss of liquor from a rupture in the fetal membranes. It may also arise however when the fetus experiences chronic hypoxia since this leads to a reduction in renal perfusion and a concomitant fall in urine production. Finally, an obstruction to fetal urinary flow will also lead to oligohydramnios, with complete obstruction causing anhydramnios – the absence of any discernible liquor around the fetus. Measurement of the liquor volume is therefore an integral component of fetal assessment.

By convention, the depth of the amniotic pool is measured in each of the four uterine quadrants, a score of zero being recorded if the quadrant is occupied by umbilical cord. The "amniotic fluid index" is given as the sum of these four values, and should be between 8 and 18 cm at full term.

The placenta

Heavy bleeding from the placental site in the second or third trimester of pregnancy jeopardises the life both of the developing fetus and its mother. The two leading causes of clinically significant haemorrhage are:

- placenta praevia
- placental abruption.

Classically, bleeding associated with placenta praevia is painless and the woman's abdomen remains soft on palpation. In contrast, placental abruption is associated with abdominal pain, the abdomen is tender, and the fetus may be difficult to palpate through a tonically contracted uterine wall. These features are however unreliable and differentiation between the two conditions frequently rests with ultrasound.

The placenta appears as a mottled, echo dense organ on ultrasound scanning. In most cases, an abdominal transducer will localise the placenta to the anterior or posterior wall of the uterus, or to its fundus. When the leading edge of the placenta lies low in the uterine cavity however, its proximity to the internal cervical os should be measured. This will allow the operator to identify the presence and severity of placental praevia and to plan for delivery if the health of the woman or fetus is compromised by bleeding.

TV scanning is known to be more accurate than abdominal scanning in measuring the distance of the placenta from the os.[3]

As an alternative, there is some evidence to support the use of translabial ultrasound in the diagnosis of placenta praevia, although this technique is less widely practised.

Since clotted blood exhibits echogenicity similar to that of placental tissue, the diagnosis of placental abruption rests on clinical history and physical examination. Occasionally however the diagnosis can be confirmed by ultrasound, for example when a large sonolucent fresh haemorrhage is identified within the substance of the placenta or at the placental edge. The management of suspected abruption, however, should not be influenced by a negative sonographic scan.

Intrapartum care

Labour is the process of progressive cervical dilatation and descent of the fetus through the genital tract. Although the role of ultrasound scanning in intrapartum care is generally poorly defined, recent evidence suggests that it can help the clinician to deal with a number of common clinical problems.

Preterm labour

For most women, labour establishes spontaneously at full term, between 38 and 42 weeks' gestation. In contrast, preterm labour complicates approximately 7% of pregnancies and is the leading cause of neonatal morbidity and mortality in developed countries. In a high risk population, TV cervical assessment in the second trimester of pregnancy may be a useful screening tool for future preterm labour since the length of the cervix at this time is inversely proportional to the likelihood of eventual preterm delivery. In contrast, the evaluation of a woman who has symptoms suggestive of preterm labour at the time of presentation to hospital remains problematic. Speculum and digital examination of the cervix is known to be unreliable in predicting preterm delivery, even in the presence of discernible uterine contractions. The findings of a short cervix, cervical dilatation of over 1 cm, and bulging of the membranes on abdominal or transvaginal[4] ultrasound are strongly suggestive of imminent or active labour however. These features may assist the clinician in determining the need for steroid therapy and treatment to abolish contractions.

Fetal presentation in labour

In labour, the leading fetal part to enter the maternal pelvis is usually its head. In 3% of cases at full term however, the fetus presents by the breech. Furthermore, the diagnosis of breech presentation is often not suspected until a vaginal examination is performed in labour, since abdominal palpation alone is an unreliable diagnostic tool. In a recent multicentre, randomised controlled trial, it was found that planned

vaginal breech delivery was significantly more hazardous for a term fetus than planned caesarean section, even when vaginal delivery was carried out by an experienced clinician.[5] Following this trial, delivery by caesarean section for this indication has become commonplace.

As a result, when the emergency physician believes a labouring woman's fetus to be presenting by the breech after abdominal or vaginal examination, abdominal ultrasound assessment is now mandatory to confirm the diagnosis and to plan for safe delivery.

Scan technique

Initially, the suprapubic area is examined by ultrasound.

Systematic examination of the lower and upper uterine segments follows, allowing the clinician to obtain a transverse section through the biparietal diameter of the fetal skull, bringing into view the falx cerebri, thalami, and cavum septum pellucidum.

Finally, flexion or extension at the knees, the attitude of the head with respect to the fetal cervical spine, the site of the placenta, and the amniotic fluid index are measured.

Knowledge of these factors may assist the clinician in determining the risk associated with attempted vaginal breech delivery on a case by case basis, since some women continue to choose vaginal breech delivery rather than caesarean section.

Evidence shows that external cephalic version can be successful in up to 50% of cases, reducing the need for caesarean section. This has led the Royal College of Obstetricians and Gynaecologists to recommend its use in selected cases late in the third trimester of pregnancy. External cephalic version has also been reported in labour. Success is most likely when the presenting part is not deeply engaged in the pelvis and when the membranes remain intact. Ultrasound also assists by allowing the clinician to monitor the fetal heart rate and to confirm fetal position throughout the procedure.

One in 200 fetuses lies transversely at full term. This may be suspected after abdominal or vaginal examination in labour but once again ultrasound is required to confirm the diagnosis. Further assessment at that time allows the clinician to determine the position of the fetal spine in relation to uterine fundus, localise the placenta, and assess the amniotic fluid index. These factors may help the clinician to determine whether stabilising external cephalic version with amniotomy is safe and practicable, or whether caesarean delivery without a prior attempt at version is indicated. Both of these procedures require the attendance of an experienced obstetrician.

Malposition

When fetal heart rate abnormalities such as prolonged bradycardia occur in the second stage of labour, an appropriately trained physician may consider effecting vaginal delivery by ventouse. Complications such as intracranial or retinal haemorrhage can arise after ventouse delivery, and failed vaginal delivery is also relatively common, with potential adverse consequences. In order to minimise these risks, the physician requires an accurate knowledge of the position of the fetal head in relation to the maternal pelvis so that the ventouse cup can be placed at its optimal position in the midline, anterior to the posterior fontanelle.

Observational work suggests that misdiagnosis of position after digital vaginal examination alone is common in labour, with an error rate of over 65%, even in experienced hands.[6] Abdominal ultrasound may have a role to play in improving the safety of instrumental vaginal delivery in this respect. Identification of the orbits is possible even when the fetal head is deeply engaged in the pelvis. The application of the ventouse may thus be guided by ultrasound, facilitating delivery and improving safety for both mother and fetus.

Approximately 1 in 500 fetuses present by the face in labour while 1 in 100 present by the brow. The diagnosis is usually suspected after digital vaginal examination, but can be confirmed by observing extension at the fetal neck on ultrasound scanning. To do this, the operator initially identifies the cervical spine, then the biparietal diameter of the head, and finally the proximity of the occiput to the spine.

Delivery of the fetus should be guided by an experienced obstetrician in these circumstances since descent of the fetal head through the maternal pelvis may be obstructed.

Retained placenta

When oxytocin, ergometrine, or a combination of the two are used in the active management of the third stage of labour, placental separation from the uterine wall usually occurs within a matter of minutes. A morbidly adherent placenta should be suspected if the third stage is not complete within thirty minutes. Manual removal of the placenta should then be contemplated, particularly if there is any associated postpartum haemorrhage.

The presence or absence of placental separation from the uterine wall can be visualised by ultrasound.[7] Manual removal of either the whole placenta or of retained individual cotyledons may then also be facilitated by abdominal ultrasound, and the presence of an empty uterine cavity confirmed at the end of the procedure.

> **Pitfalls**
> It is occasionally difficult to distinguish placental tissue from blood clot.

Summary

The use of ultrasound in the management of obstetric and gynaecological emergencies is increasing as clinicians begin to apply the technology to commonly encountered clinical events. Abdominal and TV ultrasound may be employed as diagnostic tools, to assess risk or to assist in the execution of practical procedures. Furthermore, as image resolution improves, the use of bedside ultrasound scanning as an aide to clinical practice is likely to increase in this specialty. The use of ultrasound should be restricted however to personnel who have undertaken formal training in its use, preferably with a focus on obstetric and gynaecological diseases.

References

1 Sanaullah F, Moran P, Loughney AD. The role of ultrasound in intrapartum care. *BMUS Bulletin* 2002;**10**:23–7.

2 Teisala K, Heinonen PK, Punnonen R. Transvaginal ultrasound in the diagnosis and treatment of tubo-ovarian abscess. *Br J Obstet Gynaecol* 1990;**97**:178–80.

3 Lim BH, Tan CE, Smith APM, Smith NC. Transvaginal ultrasonography for the diagnosis of placenta praevia. *Lancet* 1989;**1**:444.

4 Gomez R, Galasso M, Romero R, *et al.* Ultrasonographic examination of the uterine cervix is better than cervical digital examination as a predictor of the likelihood of premature delivery in patients with preterm labor and intact membranes. *Am J Obstet Gynecol* 1994;**171**:956–64.

5 Hannah ME, Hannah WJ, Hewson WJ, *et al.* Planned caesarean section versus planned vaginal birth for breech presentation at term: a randomized multicentre trial. *Lancet* 2000;**356**:1375–83.

6 Sherer DM, Miodovnik M, Bradley KS, Langer O. Intrapartum fetal head position II: comparison between transvaginal digital examination and transabdominal ultrasound assessment during the second stage of labor. *Ultrasound Obstet Gynecol* 2002;**19**:264–8.

7 Herman A, Weinraub Z, Bukovsky, I *et al.* Dynamic ultrasonographic imaging of the third stage of labour: new perspectives into third stage mechanisms. *Am J Obstet Gynecol* 1993;**168**:1496–9.

Further reading

Chudleigh P. Early pregnancy and complications of early pregnancy. In: Chudleigh P, Pearce MJ. eds. *Obstetric Ultrasound*. London: Churchill Livingstone, 1999.

Introduction and Key Findings. In: Lewis G. ed. *Why Mothers Die 1997–1999: The Confidential Enquiries into Maternal Deaths in the United Kingdom*. London: RCOG Press, 2001.

Whittle MJ, Chitty LS, Neilson JP, *et al* for the Working Party of the Royal College of Obstetricians and Gynaecologists. In: *Routine ultrasound screening in pregnancy. Protocol, standards and training*. London: RCOG Press, 2000.

10 Soft tissue ultrasound

ROBERT COOPER, DOMINIC BARRON

> *Objectives*
> Review soft tissue ultrasound with an emphasis on:
> - equipment, training and quality issues
> - strengths and weaknesses of the modality
> - normal tissue appearances including artefacts
> - tendon ruptures and tendinosis
> - muscle injuries
> - foreign bodies

Introduction

Soft tissue musculoskeletal ultrasound is probably the most rapidly developing area of sonography. Over the last 10 years ultrasound has spread from imaging of large superficial tendons, for rupture or gross tendinosis, to assessment of the full range of accessible musculoskeletal structures. Each of the applications and body areas has its own learning curve and even a dedicated musculoskeletal radiologist is unlikely to have a repertoire which encompasses them all. The aim of this chapter is to prime potential sonographers in the issues surrounding the topic and provide some practical general principles, before a selective coverage of potential emergency indications for soft tissue ultrasound.

General considerations

There are unlikely to be many doctors who would dispute that the needs of patients should be the starting point for the development of clinical practice, but frequently the reality is different; it is the availability of funds for equipment that often drives the process. Three questions should be addressed first.

1   What do we need to image?
2   When do we need to image?
3   Who should do the imaging?

The answers to these questions are likely to be different in the musculoskeletal clinic, with less acute problems and the opportunity for follow up or additional imaging, than in the emergency department where immediate diagnosis of acute soft issue disruption allowing early definitive treatment is required. The patient may best be served by a clinician who has a small repertoire of examinations in which they can demonstrate and maintain competence but who, when a clinical problem arises that requires imaging outside this, will refer on.

Training

Musculoskeletal ultrasound is one of the most difficult techniques to master because of the difficulty in developing the hand/eye co-ordination that is required, relearning detailed cross sectional anatomy, and understanding pathological appearances and their mimics.

High quality courses in musculoskeletal ultrasound are available which provide a good introduction to the scope and skills of the modality, but practical supervised scanning experience is often difficult to obtain. Many clinicians start out gaining experience by trial and error, either losing confidence and stopping, or making diagnostic errors. It is important to appreciate in this context that, unlike x-ray films or MRI scans, ultrasound images that are printed or recorded on video tape are of very little diagnostic value when reviewed retrospectively, making the technique extremely operator dependent.

A full history, clinical examination, and the development of a differential diagnosis is essential, firstly to ensure that the correct imaging modality is chosen, and secondly because ultrasound is a very focussed technique. Examination of a whole limb would be prohibitively time consuming! Although following the confirmation or rejection of the clinical diagnosis no further steps may be necessary, it is important to be aware of the limitations of the modality and alternative imaging modalities. Lack of this knowledge may result in inappropriate use of ultrasound and misdiagnosis.

Audit and quality assurance

Regular audit should be an integral part of clinical practice. However in reality this may prove to be much more difficult to carry out. The main difficulty is in obtaining reliable follow up as the acute trauma population is a transient one, and unless they re-attend at the same hospital it may be assumed that they have been treated appropriately, which is not always the case.

When patients remain within the hospital setting it is not always possible to obtain reliable feedback unless the patient either has definitive surgery or alternative imaging which unequivocally demonstrates the underlying pathology.

Equipment

The past 10 years has seen a quantum leap forward in ultrasound technology as a result of the huge increase in computing power and development of high resolution probes. Equipment costs have fallen as image quality has improved.

There are two main types of machines: general purpose and dedicated musculoskeletal. General purpose machines vary from large, high end equipment that is trolley based and produces the best quality soft tissue imaging to small portable scanners that, while they may be acceptable for line placement or abdominal imaging, are unsuitable for most musculoskeletal work. High and mid-range modern equipment while suitable is cumbersome and relatively expensive. At present there are two dedicated musculoskeletal machines, one trolley based and the other portable, both of which produce good image quality. Portability is superficially an attractive prospect but there are advantages of mounting such equipment on a trolley; equipment such as printers can be accommodated, the delicate machine and its probes protected from accidental damage, and lastly it may be more convenient for the operator to use. We would strongly advise that expert opinion should be sought before purchase decisions are made.

Some images should be retained. The cheapest ways of doing this are thermal paper copy or VHS tape although the image quality is poor and degrades over time. Laser printed hard copy images are better but the printer and consumables are expensive. CD/DVD writers or digital video equipment allow for good quality data storage but impose limits on access. Consideration should be given to storage of the images and data protection laws.

General principles of soft tissue ultrasound imaging

Although there has been coverage of the technical aspects of ultrasound in earlier chapters it is of such importance in understanding musculoskeletal

images that key aspects will be recounted initially. Sound is both produced and the echoes detected by a series of crystals within the probe. High frequency sound produces images of the best quality and frequencies around 10 MHz are required. Linear probes are essential for musculoskeletal scanning, and a small footprint probe is helpful for small structures such as fingers. Unfortunately high frequency sound is also attenuated more easily which restricts optimum image quality to superficial structures.

Prior to scanning it is necessary to select the settings, often referred to as presets, that allow the optimum image processing for musculoskeletal tissues. Probes focus the ultrasound beam at one or more depths in the tissue, and to obtain the best image these "focal zones" should be adjusted to coincide with the level of the structures imaged. The degree to which echo signals are magnified on the screen is determined by the "gain" controls. Most machines have an overall gain that controls echoes from all depths displayed on the screen, and selective controls for different depths.

Good quality scanning necessitates a quiet and darkened environment to view the screen, suitable couch to accommodate the patient, and an ergonomic chair for the sonographer.

Diagnostic ultrasound is reflected and absorbed at the soft tissue/bone interface resulting in many articular tissues being obscured. Reverberation artefact is often seen deep to strongly reflective interfaces such as bone. Repeated reflection between the bone and the probe results in echoes that, due to the delay in being detected, are represented as arising deep in the tissues on the ultrasound screen.

Tendons and ligaments comprise parallel bundles of collagen that, oriented parallel to the probe, produce a series of bright lines. Changing the probe orientation so that the probe is at an angle to the tendon will result in more of the echoes being reflected into the tissue rather than back to the probe so that the tendon now appears to be dark. This phenomenon is known as anisotropy and is crucial to all musculoskeletal scanning (Figure 10.1A and B). Most tendons do not run parallel to the skin and as a consequence it is necessary to be continually adjusting the probe orientation in order to examine each section to ensure that dark echo poor areas are due to anisotropy and not pathology. At the edge of many structures the increasing obliquity of the soft issue interface results in so few echoes being returned to the probe that the deeper structures

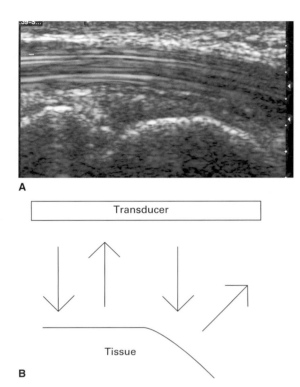

A

| Transducer |

Tissue

B

Figure 10.1 **(A)** Normal tendon demonstrating anisotropy. In the left and central portions of the image where the tendon is parallel to the probe it comprises bright lines due to the echoes being reflected straight back to the probe. On the right side of the image the tendon is oblique to the probe and echoes reflected into the adjacent soft tissues will be absorbed leading to an echo poor area of the tendon, a phenomenon known as anisotropy. **(B)** Diagrammatic representation of anisotropy.

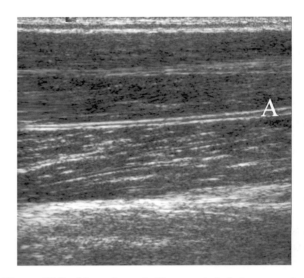

Figure 10.2 Normal muscle. The muscle belly is seen to be generally hypo-echoic with multiple linear hyperechoic lines passing through which represent the fibro-adipose septae converging upon the horizontal linear aponeurosis (A).

are not imaged at all; on the screen a shadow appears to be cast, a finding known as refractile or critical angle shadowing.

The structures being evaluated have to be carefully studied in two orthogonal planes. The bone soft tissue interface is visualised as a bright line with only noise and artefact deep to it; tendons are a series of bright lines when aligned longitudinally and bright dots when at right angles. Ligaments have a similar appearance to tendons although they are often less echo bright and, many being thin sheet like structures, may be difficult to visualise (Figure 10.1A and B).

Muscles are usually relatively dark but have a series of coarse bright lines due to the sheets of connective tissue that enclose the neurovascular supply and form the tendon insertions; in addition there are finer lines present that probably result from echoes from the muscle fibres themselves (Figure 10.2).

Fluid filled structures vary in appearance depending on the contents and the nature of the structure. Most fluid is echo poor and/or may be compressible.

Articular cartilage is very echo poor. The presence of adjacent joint fluid will produce an echo bright line between fluid and cartilage. Only a small proportion of the articular cartilage of any joint can be visualised due to the adjacent bone restricting ultrasound access.

Limitations

It is important to be aware of the limitations of any imaging modality and this is particularly so when one considers soft tissue ultrasound. There are significant restrictions in the structures that can be visualised. Bone may obstruct the view of many structures by blocking the ultrasound beam. Good image quality requires high frequency sound, which penetrates tissues poorly, restricting imaging to the first few centimetres. Both these limitations are illustrated by the knee, where although the collateral ligaments, patellar and quadriceps tendons are well visualised, the menisci, cruciate ligaments, and articular cartilage cannot be reliably assessed, making ultrasound an inappropriate method of assessing internal derangement.

Since the image is built up as a result of attenuation and echo production within tissue and the relative differences between these tissues rather than their chemical composition, as is the case in MRI, the same type of tissue may appear quite different in different patients and in different locations. One good example of this is adipose tissue, which may appear to be echo bright or echo poor, and to have different internal echo patterns depending on the patient and the anatomical location.

Knowledge of anatomy is a prerequisite to demonstration of pathology. Ultrasound poses particular problems here as, unlike MR or CT where an atlas can be consulted at leisure, the cross sectional anatomy has to be understood in real time. This is exacerbated in musculoskeletal imaging as the structures are complex and the field of view limited. Some high specification machines now allow extended field of view image reconstruction. By moving the probe over the skin in a continuous movement the scanner can produce a still image covering a large area.

The dynamic real time nature of ultrasound is often cited, but it is important to be aware that image quality falls during movement, and that in many joint positions it may not be possible to obtain any diagnostic image. An inexperienced sonographer may be unaware of absent structures. An example would be the missing rotator tendon following a retracted tear. Comparison with the contra-lateral side is often advocated but asymptomatic tears and tendinosis are common.

Specific applications

Acute tendon and ligament injuries

Tendon ruptures usually follow indirect trauma in middle aged patients. It is generally accepted that the great majority occur in tendons that are weakened by mechanical, degenerative, inflammatory, or drug induced pathology.[1] Though there are a large number of tendons that may be affected, large superficial tendons are easiest to assess sonographically and accurate diagnosis is more important in acute management.

Achilles tendon ruptures are most commonly sports related, presenting with sudden severe pain and impairment of ankle plantar flexion. Clinical examination may reveal a palpable gap in the tendon. Despite this, clinical assessment may be difficult in the acute setting, and not all patients with a classical history have a complete tear. Although the tear may be at the musculotendinous junction or the calcaneal insertion, the great majority are in the mid portion of the tendon, a distribution that may reflect preexisting tendinosis (Figure 10.3A and B). Acutely there should be a clear discontinuity in the tendon with the gap filled by haemorrhage. The

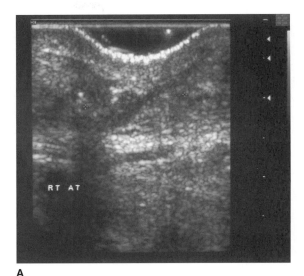

A

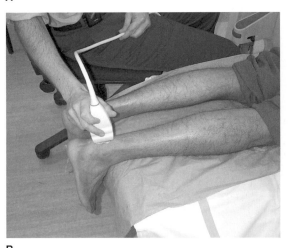

B

Figure 10.3 **(A)** Achilles' tendon rupture. There is a gap between the tendon ends marked with the two small crosses. Note the presence of refractile shadowing that helps to mark the ends of the tendon. **(B)** Probe position to examine the Achilles' tendon.

tendon ends are often defined by the presence of refractile shadowing.[2] The adjacent tendon will appear thickened and of reduced echogenicity. Important information to elicit includes the presence of a complete tear, the size of the gap between the tendon ends, and the presence of an intact Plantaris tendon. The Plantaris tendon is an accessory structure that is found superficial to the Achilles' tendon and can be utilised surgically as a graft. Scanning during passive ankle movement may help by demonstrating movement of the tendon ends, or to confirm the presence of fluid in the gap. As the haematoma becomes more organised granulation tissue and eventually scar tissue form making assessment of the tear progressively more difficult.

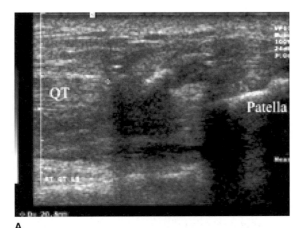

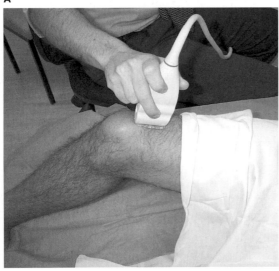

Figure 10.4 **(A)** Quadriceps tendon rupture. **(B)** Probe position to examine the quadriceps tendon.

Ruptures of the quadriceps and patellar tendons more commonly result from falls and occur in an older age group. Clinical manifestations include the presence of a gap in the tendon and loss of active extension, although such features can be misleading and there is patient benefit in an accurate and prompt diagnosis.[3] Most of these injuries are located at the distal quadriceps or proximal patellar tendon and are managed by surgical repair (Figure 10.4A and B).

Distal biceps tendon ruptures may be repaired in younger patients if the diagnosis is made sufficiently early. Since the tendon passes deep towards its insertion on the radial tuberosity at an oblique angle it can be a very difficult structure to image due to anisotropy. Our preference is for the use of MRI. Triceps tendon ruptures are rare but should be easily diagnosed acutely with ultrasound.

Although the long tendons in the foot may rupture acutely such an injury is likely to be preceded by tendon dysfunction and acute diagnosis is not usually such an important consideration.

The role of ultrasound in imaging ligament rupture is relatively restricted. Knee collateral ligaments are well visualised but since their injury is associated with damage to the menisci and cruciate ligaments which are not, MR is the preferred imaging modality. The skilled sonographer can usually demonstrate the lateral collateral ligaments of the ankle but the accuracy and role of imaging in the management of inversion injuries has yet to be determined. In the elbow radial and ulna collateral ligaments can also be imaged though further research is needed to determine the accuracy of the technique. Ultrasound can diagnose ulna collateral ligament ruptures of the thumb though the technique is outside the scope of this text.

Ligaments are of similar appearance to tendons being of similar composition but are more slender and usually less echogenic. Partial tears result in thickening and a relatively echo poor appearance. Full thickness tears are more difficult to visualise and stressing the ligament is often helpful.

Muscle/musculotendinous injuries

Ultrasound is the preferred method for imaging muscle injuries as plain radiography, scintigraphy, and computed tomography are all very limited in their ability to define muscle structure and associated pathology. MRI, although it is very sensitive for muscle injuries, does not have the same resolution as ultrasound and as a result of its water sensitivity; it tends to overestimate the extent of any injury.[4]

An appreciation of normal muscle sonographic appearance is the key to understanding muscle injury. Muscle is hypo-echoic in appearance in both longitudinal and transverse planes. Multiple hyperechoic lines can be seen to lie within the muscle representing the fibro-adipose septae, which converge upon the aponeurosis to give a herringbone like appearance (Figure 10.2). The aponeurosis blends into the tendon. The attachment of the muscle into the tendon is an essential structure to recognise as the majority of muscle tears, in the adult, occur at this point as this is the weakest part of the bone-tendon-muscle chain.

A distraction force secondary to a sudden muscular contraction causes most muscle tears.

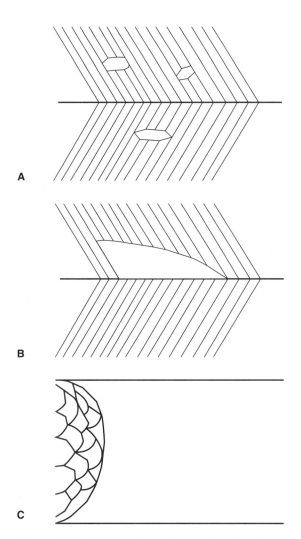

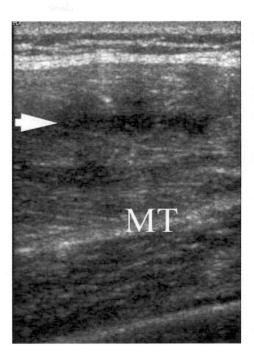

Figure 10.6 Rectus femoris muscle type 2 tear. Longitudinal image demonstrating disruption of the muscle fibres (arrow) adjacent to the myotendinous junction (MT).

Figure 10.5 **(A)** Type 1 muscle tear. The line diagram shows the "cyst-like" disruption of multiple septae. **(B)** Type 2 muscle tear. The diagram shows the more extensive muscle disruption centred around the myotendinous junction although the muscle is not completely torn. **(C)** Type 3 muscle tear. There is complete disruption of the muscle with retraction of the end and bunching of the fibres.

These are classically seen in athletes with the lower limb more commonly being affected, notably the rectus femoris, hamstrings, soleus, and gastrocnemii.

Tears can be classified into three major groups as described by Peetrons and Sintzoff.[5]

Grade 1 elongation injury

This is when the muscle has been stretched beyond its normal elasticity with resultant myofibrillar disruption. By definition, this involves less than 5% of the muscle belly and ultrasound shows multiple small hypo-echoic cavities (Figure 10.5A).

Grade 2 partial rupture

This is a more extensive injury with greater than 5% of the muscle involved, but less than the full cross-sectional area. The myotendinous junction is classically affected as described above and appears as muscle discontinuity with septal disruption. The gap between muscle fibres is filled by haematoma (Figures 10.5B and 10.6).

Grade 3 complete rupture

There is usually a clearly defined cavity between the separated ends, and the bunching of the retracted muscle ends can be readily identified (Figure 10.5C). Ultrasound has two main advantages over MRI in these injuries; it accurately estimates the degree of involvement and provides an accessible method of following the injury up. This is particularly important as it can take up to 16 weeks for healing to occur in uncomplicated cases. When this is not occurring, the follow-up scans will provide excellent delineation of the development of complications such as infection, fibrosis, or cyst formation.

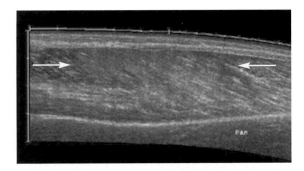

Figure 10.7 Muscle contusion. Longitudinal extended field of view image vastus lateralis muscle. Ill-defined increased echogenicity is present between the two arrows.

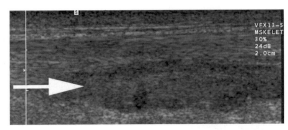

A

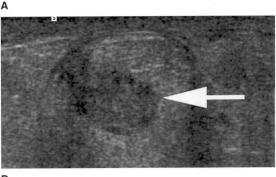

B

Figure 10.8 Achilles' tendinosis. **(A)** Longitudinal and **(B)** transverse images. There is thickening of the tendon, loss of the normal echo pattern (see figure 10.1) affecting the deep part of the tendon in this case (arrows).

The last consideration with these injuries is to reassess them once the injury has settled. This is to ensure that there is not an underlying cause for the initial tear such as a sarcoma, which would be masked at the initial scans and only become apparent once healing has occurred.[6]

Blunt muscle injury and haematomas

This group of injuries is caused by direct compressive trauma as opposed to the distraction that produces muscle tears. This is important as the nature of the injury is therefore very different from a muscle tear. Haematomas as indicated above are also seen with distraction injuries.

Haematomas can present as anything from a subtle change in echo texture of the affected muscle through to a large fluid collection (Figure 10.7). The key to diagnosis is a good clinical history and examination leading the sonographer to careful interrogation of the affected area. Gentle compression of the injured muscle will reproduce the symptoms, guiding the sonographer to the injured region. It is important to be guided by the clinical findings because a careful ultrasound examination of a large muscle group such as the quadriceps would take a prohibitively long time due to the limited field of view offered by the transducer.

Although extensive injuries are easily identified, the more subtle injuries may only become apparent by comparing the echo texture of the affected area with an appropriate comparator, such as the same muscle group on the opposite limb.

Sonographic appearances are dependent upon the time after injury. Acute haematoma appears as a well defined, hyperechoic fluid collection. After

a few hours this then becomes homogeneously hypo-echoic. This will then become more complex over the next few hours and will start to organise and eventually liquefy again.

It is very important, as with muscle ruptures, to correlate the findings with the clinical history as a large haematoma with a minor injury may well be the result of a bleeding disorder or underlying sarcoma.[6]

Chronic tendinosis/tenosynovitis

These related conditions are responsible for a large portion of the caseload in musculoskeletal medicine, and both are readily diagnosed with ultrasound.

Tendinosis is generally an overuse rather than an inflammatory condition. Although commonly sports related, it may also be seen without precipitating factors and some people are probably constitutionally predisposed to develop the condition. Aetiology is controversial but it is likely to be due to a combination of age related change and chronic micro-trauma due to tension or mechanical impingement. Disruption of the collagen structure, an increase in mucopolysaccharides and vascularity are seen at a histological level resulting in a loss of echogenicity,

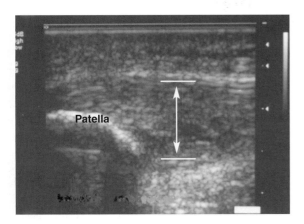

Figure 10.9 Patellar tendinosis. Longitudinal image. Proximal patella tendon and insertion into the patella. Grossly thickened and slightly heterogeneous. Similar changes are seen to that in Figure 10.8.

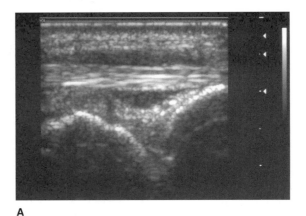

A

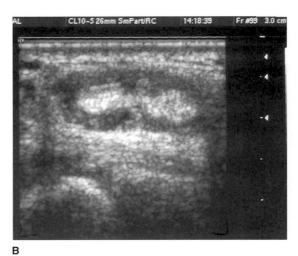

B

Figure 10.10 Tenosynovitis. **(A)** Longitudinal and **(B)** transverse images. The normal tendon is outlined by echo poor material due to thickening of the synovial lining and presence of fluid within the tendon sheath.

thickening of the tendon, and occasionally small collections of echo poor material in the tendon at sonography.[7]

The Achilles' tendon is commonly involved in participants of running sports. The mid portion of the tendon is usually affected. Sonographic changes are frequently non-uniform and often preferentially affect the superficial and medial portions of the tendon (Figure 10.8a and b). There is a second, less common type of Achilles' tendinosis which affects the distal tendon and is associated with impingement on the calcaneum.[8] Imaging abnormalities are often poorly correlated by symptoms and the contra-lateral side is frequently affected.

Patellar tendinosis affects the proximal and deep portions of the tendon preferentially and is commonly associated with sporting activity that involves jumping (Figure 10.9).[7]

Although the rotator cuff tendons are frequently affected by tendinosis and subsequent tears constituting a common indication for ultrasound examination the technique is difficult and lies beyond the scope of this text.

In the hand and foot most of the tendons have synovial sheaths. Mechanical and inflammatory conditions give rise to increased fluid and synovium within these sheaths, a condition known as tenosynovitis (Figure 10.10a and b). The peroneal and tibialis posterior tendons in the foot are commonly affected by this condition. There are often ultrasound changes within the tendon similar to those seen in tendinosis affecting other tendons, which may be associated with deformity and longitudinal tendon splitting.[9]

Foreign bodies

Although metallic foreign bodies can be readily localised by radiographs, many foreign bodies are small glass fragments which are difficult to identify or radiolucent organic material such as thorns and wood splinters. Retained foreign bodies lead to discomfort and infection. This is not just a frequent clinical problem but gives rise to medicolegal concern. Ultrasound has been demonstrated to be accurate in identification of such bodies, allows skin marking prior to surgical intervention and localisation with respect to other soft tissue structures.[10]

Since high spatial resolution is required and as foreign bodies are generally superficial, high frequency probes are required. The feet, hands, and fingers are most commonly affected so a small footprint probe is to be preferred. Glass and metal bodies being strong reflectors are readily

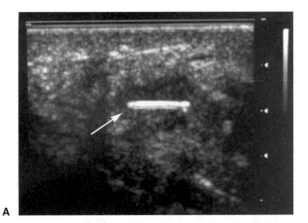

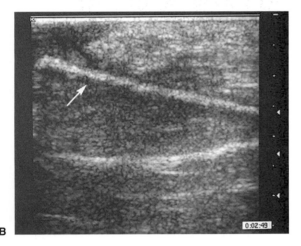

Figure 10.11 Foreign body. **(A)** Glass foreign body. Small highly echogenic with posterior acoustic shadowing. **(B)** Wooden splinter. Although less echogenic, clearly identified. Note the surrounding fluid/granulation tissue in both cases, which are several weeks old.

visualised as echo bright objects (Figure 10.11A). They often produce reverberation artefact resulting in a "comet tail" appearance. Wooden splinters and thorns having different acoustic properties are less echo bright (Figure 10.11B). Organic material produces an inflammatory reaction after a few days giving an echo poor halo that helps greatly in localisation. Wood becomes less echogenic and eventually will disappear although this process may take many months and the immunological response may produce a foreign body granuloma. All foreign bodies, but particularly metal or glass objects, have the potential to migrate.

The presence, number, size, and depth of the foreign body and its relation to bony and soft tissue structures should be described. Skin marking should be utilised if possible.

Summary

An emergency physician given basic training may be expected to diagnose most acute large tendon ruptures and some of the commoner musculoskeletal conditions. Ultrasound potentially offers a huge scope for the diagnosis of soft tissue musculoskeletal disorders but this diversity and the long learning curves associated with many of the different body areas pose numerous pitfalls for the unwary. We would commend concentration on developing a limited set of ultrasound competencies tailored to the demands of the service. Systems need to be in place to ensure that competence can be both maintained and demonstrated.

References

1 Kannus P, Jozsa L. Histological changes preceding spontaneous rupture. *J Bone Joint Surg Am* 1991; **73**(10):1507.

2 Maffulli N, Dymond NP, Capasso G. Ultrasound findings in subcutaneuos rupture of the Achilles' tendon. *J Sports Med Phys Fitness* 1989;**29**:365–8.

3 Bianchi S, Zwass A, Abdelwahab IF, Banderali A. Diagnosis of tears of the quadriceps tendon of the knee: value of sonography. *Am J Roentgenol* 1994; **162**:1137–40.

4 Takebayashi S, Takasawa H, Banzai Y, *et al.* Sonographic findings in muscle strain injury: clinical and MR imaging correlation. *J Ultrasound Med* 1995;**14**:899–905.

5 Peetrons P, Sintzoff S. Les accidents du membre inferieur chez les sportifs: Integration des differents modes d'imagerie (abstract). *J Francophone Radiol* 1987.

6 Muscolo DL, Ayerza MA, Makino A, Costs-Paz M, Aponte-Tinao LA. Tumors about the knee misdiagnosed as athletic injuries. *J Bone Joint Surg Am* 2003;**95**A(7):1209–14.

7 Khan KM, Bonar F, Desmond PM, *et al.* Patellar tendinosis: Findings at histolopathologic examination, US, and MR imaging. *Radiology* 1996;**200**: 821–7.

8 Gibbon WW, Cooper JR, Radcliffe GS. Distribution of sonographically detected tendon abnormalities in patients with a clinical diagnosis of chronic Achilles tendinosis. *J Clin Ultrasound* 2000; **28**(2):61–6.

9 Miller SD, Van Holsbeeck M, Boruta PM, Wu KK, Katcherian DA. Ultrasound in the diagnosis of tenosynovitis of the posterior tibial tendon *J Clin Ultrasound* 1990;**18**:114–6.

10 Crawford R, Matheson AB. Clinical value of ultrasonography in the detection and removal of radiolucent foreign bodies. *Injury* 1989;**20**:341–3.

Further reading

Holsbeck MT, Introcasso JH, eds. *Musculoskeletal Ultrasound*. 2nd ed. St Louis: Mosby, 2001.

Gibbon WW. *Musculoskeletal Ultrasound: The Essentials*. London: Greenwich Medical Media, 1996.

Courses

Skills Course in Musculoskeletal Ultrasound, Oxford. Director Dr D Wilson, Department of Radiology, Nuffield Orthopaedic Centre, Headington, Oxford, OX3 7LD.

British Musculoskeletal Ultrasound Course. Details from British Society of Skeletal Radiologists. www.bssr.org.uk

Acknowledgements

Dr A Grainger (Department of Musculoskeletal Radiology, Leeds Teaching Hospitals, UK) for providing many of the ultrasound images.

11 Ultrasound for bony trauma

ADAM BROOKS, JAMES L WILLIAMS

Objectives
- To introduce the concept of ultrasound (US) for the detection of bony injury
- To discuss the US technique for bony injury evaluation
- To review the current and potential applications of US in fracture detection

Table 11.1 Ultrasound sensitivity and specificity for bony trauma

Location	Sensitivity %	Specificity %
Forearm/arm	92	100
Femur	83	100
Tibia/fibula	83	100
Hand/foot	50	100

From Dulchavsky *et al. J Trauma* 2002;**53(1)**:28–32

Introduction

The development of robust ultrasound machines that are hand portable has made this technology increasingly available to emergency physicians and surgeons at the bedside. The value of hand held ultrasound has been proven in the evaluation of abdominal and thoracic trauma and recently its utility has been assessed in the diagnosis of extremity bony injury. Whilst this technique offers the theoretical advantage in urban hospitals of rapid assessment and initiation of management for long bone injuries, its use is currently most suited to specific anatomical locations and children, where conventional radiographic techniques are occasionally less reliable. It is also useful in specific austere environments such as on military deployment. It is in these situations where the introduction of hand-carried, ultrasound assessment of bony injury presents real advantages.

Imaging bony injury

Fractures of the extremities occur commonly following blunt trauma. Clinical examination and plain radiography are the mainstay of diagnosis as they enable the diagnosis to be made and a management plan formulated depending partly on fracture configuration. In certain circumstances other imaging modalities such as computerised tomography, magnetic resonance imaging, and scintography are used when plain radiographs are inadequate. These modalities are dependent on large, expensive machines to produce the images and skilled radiological personnel to interpret them. Ultrasound has the advantage of being light, portable, and relatively cheap and can be used by non-medical personnel with minimal training.[1] In a cadaver study, fractures were detectable by ultrasound

as long as the cortical interruptions were not less than 1 mm.[1,2] Dulchavsky *et al* undertook a prospective blinded study comparing extremity ultrasound by trained technicians to radiographs for the diagnosis of limb fractures. They demonstrated that the technique was sensitive and specific with an overall accuracy of 94%. Evaluation of the long bones was excellent, however they found that technical issues with the probe reduced the sensitivity of the ultrasound assessment of injury in the hands and feet (see Table 11.1).

Specific anatomical locations

In certain anatomical locations plain radiographic assessment is notoriously unreliable. This has led to ultrasound being investigated as an alternative imaging modality. The role of ultrasound has been found to be most useful with sternal fractures and rib fractures, but its use has been investigated in a wide variety of other anatomical sites.

Sternal fractures

Sternal fractures occur in up to 10% of casualties who sustain significant blunt trauma to the chest. The most frequent mechanism of injury associated with sternal fracture is a motor vehicle crash where the driver is thrown forward against the steering wheel. Sternal fractures are usually diagnosed on a lateral radiograph, however occasionally these injuries may not be visible on the *x* ray film. Fenkl confirmed the feasibility of ultrasound diagnosis of sternal fracture in 16 patients with known fractures and described interruption of the cortical reflex at the point of

Table 11.2   Ultrasound versus radiography for the detection of sternal fracture

Study	Number Patients	Number Fractures	US	XR	Sens (US)	Spec (US)	Sens (XR)	Spec (XR)
Hendrich	45	16	16	15	100	100	94	97
Bitschnau	7	7	7	7	100	100	100	100
Engin	23	20	20	16	100	100	80	43
Mahlfeld	11	11	11	11	100	100	100	100

US, ultrasound; XR, x ray; Sens, sensitivity; Spec, specificity.

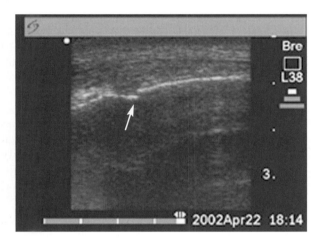

Figure 11.1   Ultrasound of sternal fracture demonstrating interruption of the cortex (arrow).

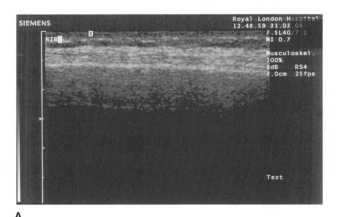

A

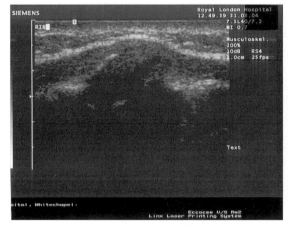

B

Figure 11.2   Ultrasound image demonstrating (**A**) normal (**B**) rib fracture.

fracture.[3] Several small studies have since compared ultrasound to x ray films in the diagnosis of sternal fracture (Table 11.2) and reported a sensitivity of 90–100% for ultrasound and several of the reports found ultrasound to be more accurate than radiographs (Figure 11.1).[4–7]

Rib fractures

The accurate diagnosis of rib fractures can be difficult from plain radiology alone. Bitschnau[4] has described the use of ultrasound in the detection of suspected rib fractures and shown that using this technique nearly twice as many rib fractures could be detected than by radiograph. Wischofer[8] investigated 21 patients with thoracic trauma, a clinical suspicion of rib fractures, and a normal chest x ray film. Ultrasound accurately diagnosed rib fractures in 16 of the patients.

Although the diagnosis of rib and sternal fractures does not necessarily always affect the immediate management of the patient, an accurate diagnosis can have significant benefits when planning longer-term management, as it can allow the level of associated morbidity to be predicted (Figure 11.2).

Other anatomical sites

The use of ultrasound has been investigated for other anatomical locations. Singh *et al*[9] investigated the use of ultrasound in injuries of the lateral complex of the ankle. They found it to be a useful adjuvant to clinical examination and postulated that it may be used to select appropriate patients for further radiological imaging. Wang[10] showed that ultrasound of the foot and ankle was able to detect occult fractures and provide important information that could potentially avoid further more complex imaging. Klinger[11] demonstrated that ultrasound could be useful in the diagnosis of orbital floor fractures and showed that ultrasound was more accurate than plain radiographs but less precise than computerised tomography. However ultrasound was less successful in diagnosing scaphoid fractures and had a sensitivity of 37% and a specificity of 61%[12] and in a study comparing ultrasound with scintography for the diagnosis of tibial stress fractures, ultrasound was only accurate in 15 out of 35 cases.[13]

Ultrasound diagnosis of extremity fractures in children

Ultrasound has been used more extensively for diagnosing extremity fractures in children than any other patient group. Plain x ray films in children can often be difficult or impossible to interpret especially if the fracture involves an area of the extremity that has not yet ossified and is therefore not visualised. As ultrasound is able to image cartilaginous structures it is ideal for imaging the developing parts of the extremity in children.

Hubner[14] compared the ultrasound examination of 163 children with 223 suspected fractures and found good correlation for fractures of the long bones of the upper and lower limbs. Ultrasound was most reliable for the detection of simple femoral and humeral diaphyseal fractures and fractures of the forearm. It was less dependable for compound injuries and fractures adjacent to joints, lesions of the small bones of the hand and foot, non-displaced epiphyseal fractures, or those with a fracture line of less than 1 mm. Kessler[15] found that ultrasound was a good imaging modality to exclude intra-articular fractures of the elbow and demonstrated that further imaging with an MRI is unnecessary when no effusion was present with ultrasound analysis. In a study investigating whether ultrasound can be reliably used to demonstrate uncomplicated wrist fractures in children, there was an absolute correlation between the ultrasound and radiographic findings.[16] Ultrasound has even been used to diagnose a fractured femur in utero.[17]

Bony US in austere environments

One of the potential applications of portable ultrasound technology is the assessment of suspected bony injury in austere or military areas. In military and austere locations radiography may not be readily available. With the increasing availability of hand held ultrasound in remote locations, attention has turned to the utility of this modality in the diagnosis of extremity trauma. Hand held ultrasound has become an asset that is routinely deployed with field hospitals and field surgical teams in operational arenas and therefore is readily available to medical personnel in these situations. Dulchavsky[1] demonstrated that even with minimal training (two hours of didatic and practical instruction) fractures could be detected with excellent accuracy and their group suggested that the technique would be appropriate for the assessment of extremity injury in space. Following this work, Kirkpatrick[18] has reported the operational use of extremity ultrasound to diagnose an ulnar fracture. Atkinson and Lennon[19] have addressed the value of extremity ultrasound as an adjunct to diagnosis and management during trauma resuscitation. They described two cases where the early ultrasound diagnosis of a femoral fracture allowed early appropriate management and analgesia.

The diagnosis of extremity fractures in the field may not necessarily influence long-term management of the fracture, but can influence appropriate limb immobilisation, timing of evacuation, and allow general but immediate predictions on outcome to be made.

Further evaluation of this area and its potential application is required. With the advent of portable, low cost systems and the growth in experience of focussed assessment with sonography for trauma (FAST) amongst emergency physicians and surgeons, the complete range of applications for ultrasound diagnosis in this field has yet to be determined.

The technique

Basics

Bony ultrasound should be performed using a high frequency 7·5–10 MHz linear transducer of appropriate dimensions to gain satisfactory images of the bony part under evaluation. Copious ultrasound gel is required. The depth should be set to maximise imaging of the cortical interface. The large acoustic impedance at the interface between bone and soft tissue causes nearly complete reflection of the ultrasound waves and this is readily visible as an unbroken, highly echogenic line. Imaging is accomplished with the transducer

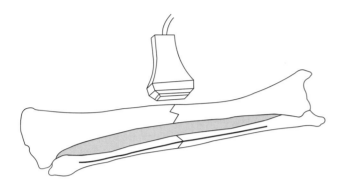

Figure 11.3 Longitudinal scanning of a tibia/fibula fracture.

scanning initially in a longitudinal plane and the cortex is assessed for irregularities, disruptions, or steps seen as interpretations and alterations in the high reflectance of the bony cortex (Figure 11.3). Suspicious areas should be further assessed with the transducer in a transverse plane. Dynamic, real-time images will allow the most accurate interpretation of cortical integrity.

Extremity ultrasound

Clinical examination and suspicion must direct the region of ultrasound assessment for extremity trauma. The dynamic ultrasound images are assessed for breaks in the echogenic cortex and soft tissue swelling (Figures 11.4 and 11.5).

Probe position

The limb is initially scanned longitudinally with the probe moved slowly across the point of maximal tenderness. Suspicious areas and regions of soft tissue swelling are then further assessed in a transverse plane.

Tips

Initial imaging of the contralateral limb provides a baseline and allows adjustment of the depth of field and gain. A smaller linear probe may be required for visualisation of bony injury in the hands or feet.

Imaging of the sternum

Ultrasound assessment should be undertaken where there is clinical suspicion of sternal injury from the mechanism of injury and appropriate tenderness on examination.

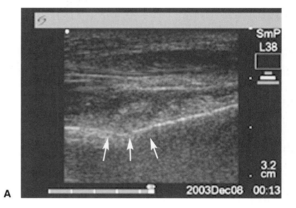

A

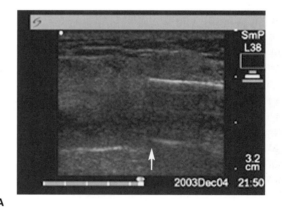

B

Figures 11.4 Ultrasound and *x* ray of distal forearm fracture. The US of the radius clearly demonstrates the angulation.

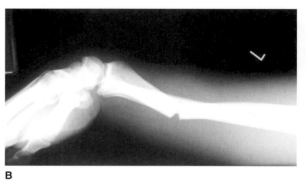

A

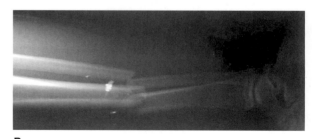

B

Figure 11.5 Ultrasound and *x* ray of lower third tibia and fibula fracture. The fractures and displacement are clearly seen on US (arrow).

Probe position

The basic technique of bony ultrasound evaluation is used with the sternum initially imaged longitudinally. The settings are adjusted so that the highly echogenic cortex is readily visible. Sternal fractures are evident as a break in this line, representative of a break in the cortex, or a step is detected in the bony outline when the fragment is displaced (Figure 11.3).

Pitfalls

Do not misinterpret the junction of the bony and xiphysternum as a fracture.

Limitations

Technical and physiological factors may limit the value of ultrasound evaluation of bony injury. Excessive swelling or obesity may degrade the quality of the image of the cortex obtained in limb trauma and it can be difficult to achieve interpretable images of the smaller bony parts with larger transducers. The examination may also be limited by patient pain and discomfort.

Clinical judgement must prevail regardless of ultrasound results, and the diagnosis of bony injury should fit the clinical picture. Extremity ultrasound, like other emergency ultrasound techniques, should be undertaken at least initially as proctored examinations with appropriate mentoring, audit of personal results, and quality assurance.

Summary

Ultrasound evaluation of extremity, rib, and sternal injury are valuable techniques that potentially present advantages especially in the austere, and military environments.

Key references

1 Dulchavsky SA, Henry SE, Moed BR. Advanced ultrasonic diagnosis of extremity trauma: the FASTER examination. *J Trauma* 2002;**53(1)**:28–32.

2 Grechenig W, Clement H, Schatz B, Klein A, Grechenig M. [Ultrasound fracture diagnosis – an experimental study]. *Biomed Tech (Berl)* 1997; **42(5)**:138–45.

3 Fenkl R, von Garrel T, Knaepler H. [Emergency diagnosis of sternum fracture with ultrasound]. *Der Unfallchirurg* 1992;**95(8)**:375–9.

4 Bitschnau R, Gehmacher O, Kopf A, Scgeier M, Mathis G. [Ultrasound diagnosis of rib and sternum fractures]. *Ultraschall Med* 1997;**18(4)**:158–61.

5 Engin G, Yekeler E, Guloglu R, Acunas B, Acunas G. US versus conventional radiography in the diagnosis of sternal fractures. *Acta Radiol* 2000; **41(3)**:296–9.

6 Hendrich C, Finkewitz U, Berner W. Diagnostic value of ultrasonography and conventional radiography for the assessment of sternal fractures. *Injury* 1995;**26(9)**:601–4.

7 Mahlfeld A, Franke J, Mahlfeld K. [Ultrasound diagnosis of sternum fractures.] *Zentralblatt Fur Chirurgie* 2001;**126(1)**:62–4.

8 Wischhofer E, Fenkl R, Blum R. [Ultrasound detection of rib fractures for verifying fracture diagnosis. A pilot project.] *Der Unfallchirurg* 1995;**98(5)**:296–300.

9 Singh A.K, Malpass TS, Walker G. Ultrasonic assessment of injuries to the lateral complex of the ankle. *Arch Emerg Med* 1990;**7(2)**:90–4.

10 Wang C.L, Shieh JY, Wang TG, Hsieh FJ. Sonographic detection of occult fractures in the foot and ankle. *J Clin Ultrasound* 1999;**27(8)**:421–5.

11 Klinger M, Danter J, Siegert R. [Ultrasound diagnosis of orbital floor fractures: an alternative to computerized tomography?] *Laryngo-Rhino-Otologie* 1996;**75(4)**:242–6.

12 Christiansen T.G, Rude C, Lauridsen KK, Christensen OM. Diagnostic value of ultrasound in scaphoid fractures. *Injury* 1991;**22(5)**:397–9.

13 Boam W.D, Miser MF, Yuill SC, Delaplain CB, Gayle EL, MacDonald DC. Comparison of ultrasound examination with bone scintiscan in the diagnosis of stress fractures. *J Am Board Fam Prac* 1996; **9(6)**:414–7.

14 Hubner U, Schlicht W, Outzen S, Barthel M, Halsband H. Ultrasound in the diagnosis of fractures in children. *J Bone Joint Surg* 2000;**82(8)**: 1170–3.

15 Kessler T, Winkler H, Weiss C, Konermann W, Gruber G. [Ultrasound diagnosis of the elbow joint in fracture of the head of the radius.] *Der Orthopade* 2002;**31(3)**:268–70.

16 Williamson D, Watura R, Cobby M. Ultrasound imaging of forearm fractures in children: a viable alternative? *J Accid Emerg Med* 2000;**17(1)**:22–4.

17 Watson NA, Ferrier GM. Diagnosis of femoral shaft fracture in pregnancy by ultrasound. *J Accid Emerg Med* 1999;**16(5)**:380–1.

18 Kirkpatrick AW, Brown R, Diebel LN, Nicolau S, Marshburn T, Dulchavsky SA. Rapid diagnosis of an ulnar fracture with portable hand-held ultrasound. *Mil Med* 2003;**168(4)**:312–3.

19 Atkinson P, Lennon R. Use of emergency department ultrasound in the diagnosis and early management of femoral fractures. *Emerg Med J* 2003;**20(4)**:395.

12 Ultrasound for venous access

RICHARD G McWILLIAMS, CHRISTOPHER BOYD

Objectives
- To discuss general principles of venous access
- To introduce the general principles of ultrasound-guided venous access
- To discuss the ultrasound anatomy of the jugular, subclavian, and femoral veins
- To introduce the methods used for ultrasound-guided puncture of central veins

General principles of venous access

Venous access has traditionally been divided into two categories, specifically central access and peripheral access. Central venous access, by definition, involves the insertion of cannulae or vascular lines into large calibre central veins. The veins typically used for central venous access are the internal jugular, subclavian, and femoral veins. A more recent development in the field of venous access is the peripherally inserted central venous catheter or PICC line. These access lines are inserted percutaneously in the upper limb but the line tip lies within a central vein, typically the superior vena cava.

Peripheral venous access describes the placement of an intravenous cannula into a vein located classically in the antecubital fossa or the dorsum of the hand. Occasionally a vein in the lower limb, usually the great saphenous vein, is used. The placement of these cannulae is outside the remit of this chapter.

Central venous catheter placement

The indications for the placement of a central venous catheter (CVC) are numerous and detailed discussion is beyond the scope of this chapter. However in broad terms access is required for drug administration, typically chemotherapy, or total parenteral nutrition, fluid administration, haemodialysis, or invasive cardiovascular monitoring purposes.

Typically, when CVCs are required for long-term access, tunnelled catheters are preferred whereas for short-term access non-tunnelled devices are used. The definition of long-term in this respect is conventionally taken as > 30 days. Many studies have shown that long-term tunnelled lines are associated with a lower rate of line infection than non-tunnelled lines although the data are not unanimous.

The choice of insertion site of a CVC depends on a number of factors including:

- indication for CVC placement
- anticipated time scale for CVC necessity
- venous anatomy of the individual patient
- presence of pre-existing catheters
- venous thrombosis or other morbidity
- CVC insertion physician preferences.

A number of studies have concluded that non-tunnelled CVCs inserted via the subclavian route are associated with a lower infection rate than those placed via the jugular route. It is however generally accepted that subclavian venous access carries a higher risk of procedural mechanical complication than jugular catheterisation.

Regardless of the site of venous access chosen, the use of full aseptic technique for CVC insertion is central to minimisation of infection. This involves the use of full barrier precautions including large skin drapes and operator gown and gloves as well as skin preparation, ideally using a chlorhexidine gluconate solution, as this has been shown to be superior in terms of reduction of line infection to other skin preparatory agents.

Traditionally the placement of long-term tunnelled CVCs was the remit of the vascular surgeon in the operating room while shorter-term catheters were more usually placed by an anaesthetist. In recent years this pattern has altered as interventional radiologists have developed services for CVC placement using image guidance techniques. The role of the anaesthetist and the intensivist in the insertion of CVCs however remains central in the setting of the operating room, intensive care unit, and high dependency unit. When inserting CVCs in these settings venous access has traditionally been established by the landmark method without any form of imaged needle guidance. The recent guidelines issued by the National Institute For Clinical Excellence (NICE) has questioned such techniques and advocates the development of skills to allow ultrasound (US) guidance of the accessing needle and the target vessel to minimise procedural iatrogenic morbidity.

General principles of ultrasound-guided venous access

There are three advantages to the use of two-dimensional greyscale imaging for venous access. Firstly, preliminary scanning allows the operator to choose the most suitable vein for puncture. Secondly, ultrasound may be used to guide the needle into the target vein. Thirdly, the guidewire may be imaged after introduction to confirm that this is within the lumen of the vein. These three advantages will now be considered in turn.

Preliminary scanning

Significant time can be saved by scanning the intended site for access before proceeding to draping and anaesthetising the area. The jugular vein is the most common site chosen for ultrasound-guided venous access. Both sides of the neck can be scanned quickly to determine if one side is more suitable for access. Reasons to choose one jugular vein over the other include the size and patency of the vein and its relationship to the carotid artery. In the majority of patients the jugular vein lies anterolateral to the carotid artery, however, in a small percentage of patients the jugular vein is anterior to the carotid artery and in this location inadvertent arterial puncture is more likely. When all things are equal then the right internal jugular is the preferred vein, as the avenue to the superior vena cava is straighter resulting in less difficulty and complications from catheter access.

The operator must be able to distinguish the jugular vein from the carotid artery. This distinction relies on a knowledge of the standard anatomical relationships and also on the shape and compressibility of the vein. The carotid artery is usually nearly circular whereas the jugular has a more variable shape (Figure 12.1). More important in distinguishing the artery from the vein is the response to compression of the overlying soft tissues with the ultrasound transducer. The jugular vein readily compresses with light pressure whereas the carotid artery,

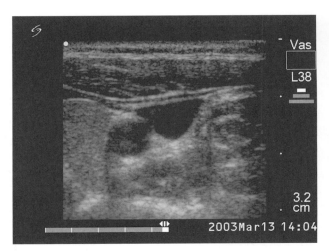

Figure 12.1   Transverse US of neck showing internal jugular vein (triangular) and CCA (circular).

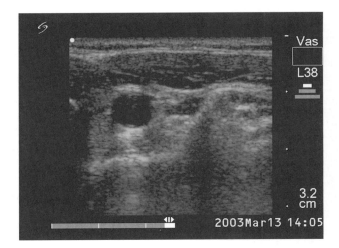

Figure 12.2   Internal jugular vein compression after pressure applied by operator.

which is more pressurised, retains its shape. The corollary of this is that if the operator presses inadvertently too heavily on the skin with the ultrasound probe, then he may mistakenly think that the jugular vein is occluded (Figure 12.2). The technique employed during scanning can minimise the potential for a false diagnosis of jugular vein occlusion. It is important to rest a finger or the ulnar border of the scanning hand on the neck to provide a point of counter-pressure (Figure 12.3). This ensures stability of the probe, which is also essential for needle guidance with ultrasound.

Spectral Doppler ultrasound may be used, if available, to distinguish the carotid artery from the jugular vein. Spectral Doppler shows

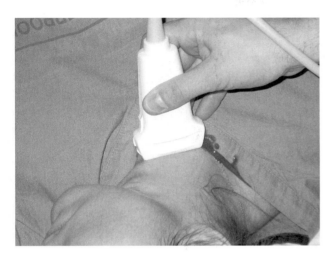

Figure 12.3 Correct technique for holding the probe ensuring visualisation of scanhead and access site on skin.

graphically how the Doppler frequency shift varies with time and the spiky arterial waveform is markedly different from the more uniform venous waveform. There will however be some variation in the venous waveform due to respiration and transmitted pulsation from the adjacent artery.

In practice, Doppler imaging is rarely necessary for jugular venous or femoral venous access as the compressibility of the vein on greyscale imaging allows artery and vein to be distinguished. Doppler ultrasound can be helpful for subclavian venous access where compression is sometimes more difficult as the vessels are at a greater depth from the skin surface.

Preliminary scanning also involves adjusting the machine settings to optimise the image prior to needle puncture. If there is a choice of ultrasound probes then a linear probe with a small footprint (size of the scanhead) is preferred. There are likely to be programmed pre-sets that automatically adjust many of the machine variables. If there is a pre-set labelled "veins" then this should be chosen. Further adjustments to the gain and depth may be made. The gain should be set quite low so that the echogenic needle tip will stand out against the surrounding soft tissue. The depth is ideally varied to show all of the target vein and the important surrounding structures, usually the companion artery. An important step after or before this is to make certain that the controls have been adjusted to switch off or delay the automatic shut-off that occurs with many machines if they are not used for a variable number of minutes. It can be very

frustrating to set the machine up ideally but find that it automatically powers down just after proceeding to sterilise the probe and prepare the operative field.

If a biopsy attachment is to be used then it is also necessary to switch on the on-screen needle guidelines. The probe should at this stage be sterilised with the use of a sterile probe cover that contains some ultrasound gel.

Needle guidance

This involves following the needle through the scan plane into the target vessel. The correct use of US allows visualisation of the target vein for CVC insertion together with imaging of the access needle as it traverses the tissues from skin to vein. This constitutes real-time US needle guidance and is the technique advocated by NICE. It differs from the markedly inferior US-premapping technique, which comprises US interrogation of the tissues at the proposed site of venous access, identification of the target vein, then "blind" non-guided venous puncture.

Needle guidance under US imaging is not a complex technique but it is a different skill to venous access using the landmark technique. Ultrasound in unskilled hands may make a negative contribution and increase the risks of the procedure. During the procedure there is temporary separation of visual and motor axes, and it is during these periods when the operator is looking at the ultrasound monitor that the hands may advance the needle in an inappropriate direction to an inappropriate depth. The separation of the visual and motor axes can be minimised by siting the ultrasound monitor as close to and nearly in line with the operative field (Figure 12.4).

It is crucial to understand that the ultrasound beam is focussed by the transducer into a narrow beam that is only 1 or 2 mm wide (Figure 12.5). This is disappointing to many people who start to use ultrasound. Despite the width of the transducer, which may be of the order of 1 cm, the actual US beam width will be much narrower. The practical consequence of this is that the needle tip will only be seen when it is within this very narrow beam width.

There are two methods of needle guidance. The first method is known as the freehand technique and this is the method most commonly used. The second method involves the use of external biopsy guides or biopsy probes that limit the path

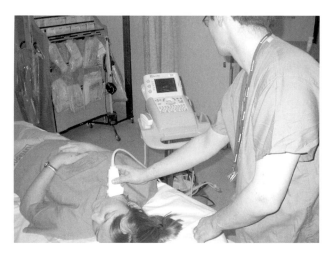

Figure 12.4 Correct positioning of operator and US screen for maximum efficiency.

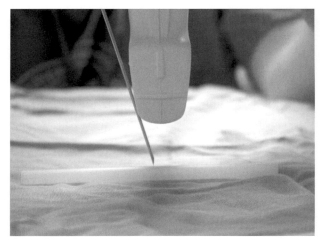

Figure 12.6 Steep angle of needle passage to keep needle in scan plane.

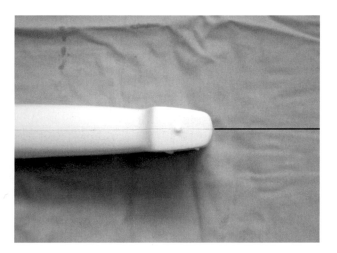

Figure 12.5 Narrow US beam width.

of the needle which should pass through the image within the on-screen guidelines.

Freehand targeting may be performed either with transverse or longitudinal scanning. Transverse scanning is most commonly used for jugular and femoral venous access because this allows the operator to observe the vein and companion artery in the one image. A basic principle to absorb is that there is a one-to-one correspondence between the image on the monitor and the transducer. So if the jugular vein is positioned so that it lies exactly in the middle of the monitor screen then one can be certain that the vein lies beneath the middle of the transducer. The operator should hold the probe such that the hand holding the probe does not obscure the view

of the scanhead otherwise the relationship of the vein to the transducer will be difficult to appreciate (Figure 12.3).

The jugular vein typically lies 1 to 3 cm from the skin surface and is most easily punctured between the sternal and clavicular heads of the sternocleidomastoid muscle. For US-guided venous access the jugular vein is scanned in a transverse plane at this level. The probe is positioned so that the vein lies in the middle of the ultrasound screen and thus lies directly below the middle of the transducer. The transducer is held so that it is either at 90 degrees to the skin or angling slightly upwards. The needle is then passed through the skin just cephalad to the transducer and held at a steep angle. The steep angle allows the needle tip to be seen as it indents and then passes into the vein. This needle angulation (Figure 12.6) is very different to the shallower angle used for puncture using the landmark method. A shallower angle may be used but it is much more difficult to follow the needle into the vein as it is a more complex exercise in triangulation to work out where the needle tip and the scan plane will intersect. If the needle is held steeply then it is much easier for the scan plane and needle to coincide, and thus for the needle to be followed through the image plane to the vein. In practice very small movements of the probe are often necessary to allow the needle to be followed through the soft tissues into the jugular vein.

It is very common for the needle to indent the anterior wall of the vein without initially passing through the anterior wall. This is easily observed with ultrasound. The final passage of the needle

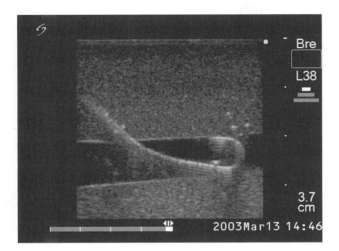

Figure 12.7 US image of wire in vessel lumen.

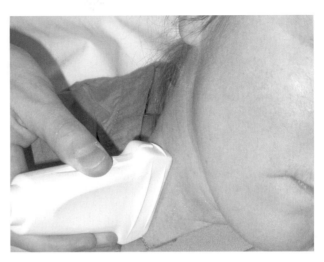

Figure 12.8 Longitudinal scanning of the internal jugular vein.

through the anterior wall of the jugular vein often requires a short darting movement of the needle to puncture rather than merely indent the vein wall. Aspiration of venous blood confirms entry to the vein lumen and this can be reinforced by ultrasound imaging of the guidewire in the vein if an over-the-wire catheter system is used (Figure 12.7).

This technique of scanning and needle puncture using transverse scanning is also used for puncturing the femoral vein.

Longitudinal freehand targeting

Here the long axis of the transducer head is in line with the long axis of the target vein. This is the method most commonly used for puncturing the axillary and subclavian veins. Jugular and femoral veins may be punctured using longitudinal rather than transverse scanning. However, longitudinal scanning often does not allow the companion artery to be seen in the same image as the vein. Also the width of many probes means that puncturing using a longitudinal approach in the neck will result in a very high point of access in the neck (Figure 12.8).

Again it must be appreciated that the ultrasound beam is focussed into a narrow beam and unless the needle is within this narrow beam then it will not be seen. The operator must also orientate the probe so that he knows where the needle will appear in the image. If the operator holds the probe wrongly and expects the needle to arrive from the left of the image when it actually arrives in the right of the image, then the needle may be inadvertently advanced too far as the operator watches the screen. This point is most easily

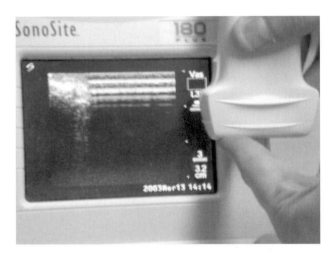

Figure 12.9 Ensuring correct transducer orientation.

appreciated when holding the transducer and scanning. The most commonly used method for orientating the probe is to touch one edge of the transducer head with a finger and see which edge of the image records this event (Figure 12.9).

The operator must now advance the needle in the same plane as the transducer and watch the needle pass through the scan plane until it indents the wall of the target vein. If the needle is not seen in the image then it is because the scan plane and the needle plane are different. It is best to look at the needle direction to determine which corrective movement is needed. A very gentle fanning movement of the transducer head may find the needle, which only needs to be minimally off line to be outside the focussed scan plane and hence not seen.

Biopsy guides

Biopsy guides may be used for both transverse and longitudinal scanning. The basic principle is that the external guide attached to the transducer restricts the path of the needle in a way that the ultrasound machine is calibrated to understand. The set-up menu of machines with guides allows these on-screen guidelines to be switched on when required. The operator must attach the biopsy guide and position the transducer so that the on-screen guidelines intersect the target vein. The depth from the guide to the target can be calculated and a needle of suitable length chosen. The needle is then advanced through the guide and can be seen in the image. It is then followed to the point of venous puncture. A good biopsy guide thus converts a three-dimensional problem with much scope for human error into a two-dimensional problem that demands that the operator stops advancing the needle when the vein is punctured.

If the needle that is chosen is very flimsy then it is possible for the needle to be diverted from the on-screen guidelines if it encounters any resistant tissues such as thick fibrous layers.

Most guides are designed for longitudinal scanning. However, external guides for transverse scanning do exist. The design of these is slightly different as the needle will not be in the scan plane for all of its path. Generally the depth of the target structure is measured and an adaptor chosen for the guide such that the needle will intersect the guide at the appropriate depth in the image plane. The further the target is from the skin surface the steeper the needle path needs to be.

Biopsy guides can be awkward and the operator must make sure that the guide and adaptor do not compromise the sterility of the procedure. The operator must also be familiar with the mechanisms for separation of the guide and needle after the vein has been accessed. It is generally best to leave the guide attached while the wire is introduced and then to dissociate the guide and needle.

Many experienced operators prefer to use a freehand approach for ultrasound-guided procedures. As ultrasound becomes adopted by more and more users it is likely that biopsy guides will be more frequently used and it may be reasonable to expect that this will lead to improvements in the reliability and ease of use of biopsy guides. A summary of the differences between freehand needle guidance and biopsy guide use is given in Table 12.2.

Table 12.1 Ultrasound differentiation of artery from vein

	Artery	Vein
Visible pulsation	Yes	No
Compressible	No	Yes
Valsalva effect	None	Dilates
Doppler trace	Pulsatile flow	Continuous flow

Guidewire scanning

Despite successful ultrasound-guided venous puncture and aspiration of venous blood, failed cannulation may still occur if the operator inadvertently advances the needle through the posterior vein wall during syringe detachment or as the guidewire is introduced. If the companion artery lies immediately deep to the vein then it is possible to advance the wire into the artery. There are reports of ultrasound users placing central lines in the carotid artery despite having seen the needle pass into the jugular vein. These mistakes can be avoided by always scanning the vein after the guidewire has been introduced. Metal is highly reflective of ultrasound and is very easily seen in both transverse and longitudinal images (Figure 12.7). The operator can confirm that the wire is running freely in the vein and inadvertent arterial catheterisation can be avoided.

Jugular venous access

The internal jugular vein (IJV) is the preferred route of CVC insertion by most interventional radiologists. The reasons for this include:

- its easy identification on US
- the relative ease of puncturing the vessel under US guidance
- the ability to visualise the common carotid artery beside the vein and thereby prevent inadvertent arterial puncture
- the relatively straight path from the IJV to the superior vena cava and right atrium.

Anatomy

The IJV begins at the base of the skull as a continuation of the sigmoid sinus as it passes through the jugular foramen. The vein lies within the carotid sheath. This is a fascial sheath that

Table 12.2 Comparison of freehand vs. needle guide for venous puncture

	Freehand	*Needle guide*
Additional cost	None	Cost of guide
Sterility	Standard precautions	Extra care due to use of guide
Target imaging	Operator dependent	Path of needle to target displayed
Surface anatomy	Can move transducer to optimise image	Transducer movement limited by guide
Anatomy around target vessel	Operator can display target vessel and other structures	Limited views due to need to keep target vessel in view
Operator skill	Requires appreciation of 2-D US image and needle control	Less operator skill needed for safe puncture
Training issues	More training needed	Less training needed
Operator flexibility	Suitable for needle guidance using any US machine	Limited skills not directly transferable to freehand technique

surrounds the IJV, the internal and common carotid arteries, and the vagus nerve. The IJV ends behind the sternoclavicular joint by joining with the subclavian vein to become the brachiocephalic vein. At its most caudal limit, just prior to its termination, the IJV lies immediately anterior to the subclavian artery. This relationship is important for low IJV puncture, as a needle passing too deep is likely to hit this artery. The IJV usually contains a valve at its point of union with the subclavian vein.

Ultrasound imaging

The IJV is best imaged in the transverse plane for CVC insertion. A useful skin landmark for transducer placement is the triangle formed by the two heads of sternocleidomastoid muscle and the clavicle as the vein typically lies deep to this anatomical triangle.

Vein identification and optimising visualisation

The IJV lies in close proximity to the common carotid artery. The artery is usually posteromedial to the artery but in some patients lies immediately posterior to the IJV. The IJV appears as an approximately circular shaped echo-poor structure and often the valve leaflets may be seen within the lumen. Several features can be used to correctly differentiate artery from vein and help assist venous puncture.

- The IJV is usually slightly irregular in shape. The artery is typically circular (Figure 12.1).
- Vein distension is improved by placing the patient with head-down tilt.
- Vein distension is improved by the use of a Valsalva manoeuvre.
- Vein is easily compressible by pressure with the transducer over the vessel. The artery is not compressible in this way (Figure 12.2).
- The artery walls are seen to oscillate with each pulse. The walls of the vein do not so move with each cardiac cycle.
- Doppler traces from within the lumen of the vein show continuous venous flow while a trace from within the artery lumen will give a typical arterial trace. (See sections on subclavial and femoral Doppler for images.)

Table 12.1 summarises the differentiating features of artery and vein.

It is important to appreciate that the amount of pressure required to compress the vein is very little and this often surprises those new to venous US scanning. The corollary of this is that if the operator scans with too much pressure on the patient it is possible to mistakenly believe that the vein is occluded or absent when it is in fact normal. This is why it is important to rest the ulnar border of the scanning hand on the patient to act as a counterbalance to the weight of the transducer to ensure light scanning.

If the patient has had previous CVC placements then the IJV may be acutely or chronically thrombosed. The presence of fresh thrombus is seen as echogenic material within the vessel lumen, which causes venous distension and prevents the normal easy venous compression with light transducer pressure. Chronic thrombosis typically results in venous obliteration with no IJV visible on US imaging.

Positioning patient and equipment

It is essential that the patient, operator, and US machine are positioned for maximum comfort and ease of procedure. The patient will be lying supine or slightly head-down tilt. The operator should typically stand at the head of the patient with the US monitor directly facing him so that there is minimal eye or body movement required to view the operation area and the US image.

US-guided IJV puncture

The puncture of the IJV is typically performed in transverse section. This permits both the target IJV and the adjacent artery to be visualised simultaneously to assist in correct venous puncture and avoid accidental arterial puncture. In the small percentage of patients in whom the jugular vein lies immediately in front of the carotid artery the needle puncture is a little more difficult as there is the risk of a two-wall vein puncture, resulting in carotid artery injury. This risk can be avoided by either directing the needle to pass in an angled path through the vein or by scanning the vein a little more laterally so that the vein and artery are separated (Figure 12.10).

After venous puncture and guidewire advancement it is usually possible to view the first 1 or 2 cm of the brachiocephalic vein by angling the transducer behind and deep to the clavicle (Figure 12.11) and thus confirm that the wire has not turned the corner into the subclavian vein as occasionally happens. If either the wire catches on the jugular valve or if it passes into the subclavian vein then the wire can be withdrawn slightly and re-advanced under ultrasound guidance.

Subclavian venous access

Ultrasound guided puncture of the subclavian vein is technically more challenging than puncture of the internal jugular vein. It is generally accepted that the procedural complication rate for subclavian venous access is greater than that for

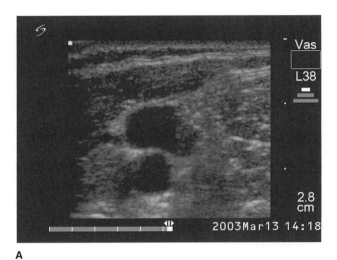

A

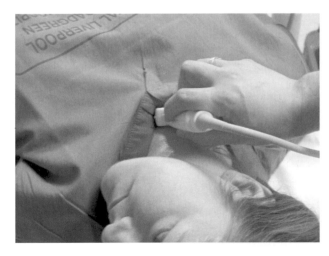

B

Figure 12.10 **(A)** IJV and CCA in same vertical plane. **(B)** Lateral scanning to separate vessels for safer puncture.

Figure 12.11 Angling transducer behind clavicle to image brachiocephalic vein.

jugular access. This is largely attributable to the close proximity of the subclavian artery and the lung apex to the subclavian vein as well as the relative difficulty of adequately imaging the vein to allow secure guided access. For these reasons most interventional radiologists choose the IJV as the preferred route of CVC insertion rather than the subclavian vein. However as previously stated there are some data indicating that non-tunnelled subclavian lines are associated with a lower infection rate than jugular lines. These factors must be balanced when deciding on the preferred site of CVC insertion.

Anatomy

The subclavian vein is a continuation of the axillary vein. It commences at the outer border of the first rib and passes medially, to end by joining the internal jugular vein to form the brachiocephalic vein posterior to the sternoclavicular joint. The subclavian artery is immediately posterior and the lung apex and its overlying pleura are immediately caudal to the vein.

Ultrasound imaging

In order to image the subclavian vein a useful approach is to commence with the transducer below and parallel to the outer half of the clavicle. In this plane the subclavian vessels are usually seen in oblique section. By rotating the transducer so that the lateral side of it is caudal to the medial side, the vessel will then be seen in longitudinal section. A 90 degree rotation from this position will show the artery and vein side-by-side in transverse section.

In reality US imaging in this way, although described as subclavian imaging, is actually imaging of the more medial portion of the axillary vein. This is because at this site the operator is imaging the vein lateral to the first rib because the overlying clavicle prohibits more medial imaging of the true subclavian vein, as it commences as the axillary vein crosses over the first rib. Therefore any US guided venous access at this site is in strict anatomical terms actually axillary venous access or axillary/subclavian vein junction venous access.

Vein identification and optimising visualisation

The principles of optimally identifying the subclavian vein and correctly differentiating it

from the companion artery are identical to those described for the internal jugular vein and differentiating it from the common carotid artery.

- The vein distension is improved by placing the patient with head-down tilt.
- Vein distension is improved by the use of a Valsalva manoeuvre.
- The vein is easily compressible by pressure with the transducer over the vessel. The artery is not compressible in this way.
- The artery walls are seen to oscillate with each pulse. The walls of the vein do not so move with each cardiac cycle.
- Doppler traces from within the lumen of the vein show continuous venous flow while a trace from within the artery lumen will give a typical arterial trace. (Figure 12.12)

Positioning patient and equipment

Before commencing the procedure it is essential to have the patient and the US machine positioned correctly for maximum ease of operation. A comfortable position with ease of access to the relevant skin area and clear view of the US monitor makes the procedure both easier and safer. A recommended position is shown in Figure 12.13. In this position the operator stands above the shoulder of the patient and the US monitor is immediately anterior to the operator so that no movement is required to alternate the gaze between the patient and the monitor. Full aseptic technique must be observed and sterile US transducer cover and sterile US gel used.

US-guided subclavian puncture

This can be done when viewing the subclavian vein in either longitudinal or transverse section. The main advantage of longitudinal imaging is that it is easier to keep the target vessel in view and watch and guide the needle into it throughout the entire course of the needle track through the intervening tissues. Additionally there is less risk of "losing" the needle tip and inadvertently passing it too deep and puncturing the pleura, which lies just deep to the vessel. When the vein has been entered check aspiration will confirm luminal needle position and a guidewire can be advanced. After this track dilation and catheter insertion are usually straightforward.

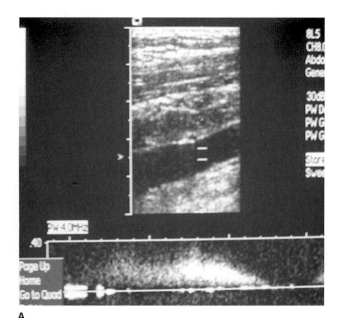

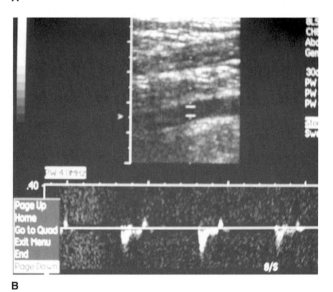

A

B

Figure 12.12 **(A)** Doppler trace of subclavian vein. **(B)** Doppler trace of subclavian artery.

Femoral venous access

The femoral venous route is most commonly used for the insertion of temporary lines for central venous access purposes. Some data indicate a higher rate of line infection with femoral access and a higher rate of deep venous thrombosis than observed when internal jugular or subclavian sites are used for CVC insertion.

Anatomy

The common femoral vein (CFV) is the vessel in which access is ideally achieved. It is formed by

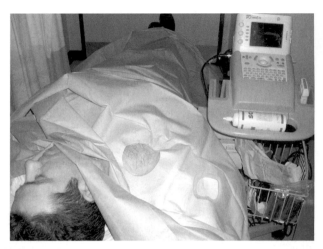

Figure 12.13 Positioning for subclavian puncture.

the union of the deep and superficial femoral veins and ends by passing behind the inguinal ligament to become the external iliac vein. The CFV has a number of tributaries but the main one for US imaging purposes is the great saphenous vein which enters the CFV on its medial side 2–3 cm caudal to the inguinal ligament. The common femoral artery (CFA) lies on the lateral side of the CFV. The vessels lie within a defined anatomical region called the femoral triangle. As well as the CFV and CFA the femoral triangle contains lymphatic vessels and the femoral nerve. A useful aide memoire to the anatomic relationships of these contents is "NAVEL" which describes the contents from lateral to medial:

Nerve – Artery – Vein – (Empty) – Lymphatics.

Ultrasound imaging

For US imaging of the CFV and guided access the simplest approach is to image the vessel in transverse section. The groin skin crease provides a useful start position for the US transducer, which is placed at 90 degrees to the long axis of the lower limb. In this position the CFV will be seen with the artery lying on its lateral side (Figure 12.14).

Vein identification and optimising visualisation

A number of useful methods are available to allow correct identification of the CFV and correct discrimination of it from the accompanying artery.

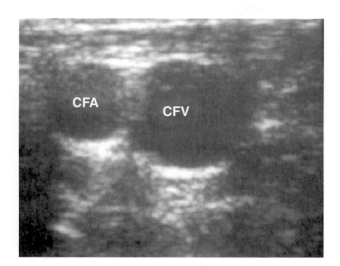

Figure 12.14   Relationship of common femoral artery and vein.

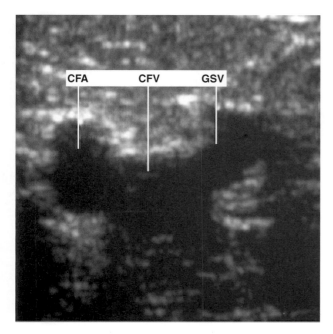

Figure 12.15   "Mickey Mouse" sign comprising common femoral artery and vein and great saphenous vein.

- Vein distension is improved by the use of a Valsalva manoeuvre.
- The artery lies lateral to the vein. Remember "NAVEL".
- The great saphenous vein enters the CFV on its medial side. This together with the artery on the lateral side gives an appearance that has been described as "The Mickey Mouse Sign" (Figure 12.15).
- The CFV is easily compressible. The artery is not.
- The walls of the artery move with the cardiac cycle. Those of the CFV do not.

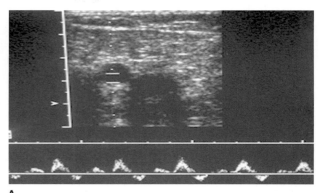

A

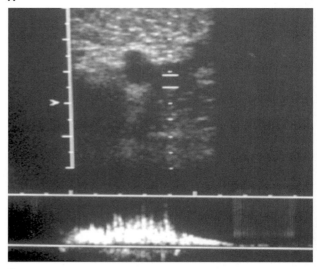

B

Figure 12.16   **(A)** Doppler trace common femoral artery. **(B)** Doppler trace common femoral vein.

- Doppler signals from the artery and the vein each show characteristic arterial and venous traces (Figure 12.16).

Positioning patient and equipment

As with other sites for CVC placement it is essential to correctly position both the patient and the equipment to be used, to maximise the ease and safety of the procedure. The operator stands beside the patient just caudal to the level of the patient groin. The US monitor is positioned on the contralateral side of the patient. An alternative position for the ultrasound is to place it on the ipsilateral side of the patient directly facing the operator. As before full patient and US aseptic preparation is required.

US-guided femoral venous puncture

US-guided access is best achieved when imaging the vessel in the transverse plane. In this respect the procedure is identical to venous access of the IJV and so will not be repeated here.

Peripheral venous access

In recent years there has been an increase in the number of peripherally inserted central lines (PICC lines) used for chemotherapy. PICC lines have several potential advantages over traditional CVCs. Firstly they can be placed in virtually any moderate-size vein in either upper limb and often can be placed without the necessity for US-guided venous puncture. Their smaller calibre and their site of insertion result in a simple insertion procedure with little attendant iatrogenic morbidity. Infection data indicate that PICC lines have a relatively low infection rate and are therefore suitable for long-term central venous access. In addition patients usually find them more cosmetically acceptable.

Although many PICC lines are inserted without US-guided venous access the use of US is to be recommended for their insertion. It allows the operator to identify the desired vein and guide the access needle into it, often with a single needle pass. In patients with poor peripheral venous access and no identifiable superficial veins US permits visualisation of deeper veins including the brachial veins, which may be used for PICC insertion. Additionally the operator can identify the brachial artery and ensure avoidance of inadvertent arterial puncture.

Anatomy

The venous drainage of the upper limb is via a deep and a superficial system. The deep system is the counterpart of the arterial system with radial and ulnar veins in the forearm that unite below the elbow to form a brachial vein, which is the dominant deep vein in the upper arm. Often there is a pair of brachial veins with one on each side of the artery. The superficial system consists of numerous channels with a dominant vein on the medial side of the limb, the basilic vein, and one on the lateral side, the cephalic vein. The basilic vein usually enters the brachial vein at mid-upper arm level while the cephalic vein extends more centrally before entering the axillary vein at approximately shoulder level.

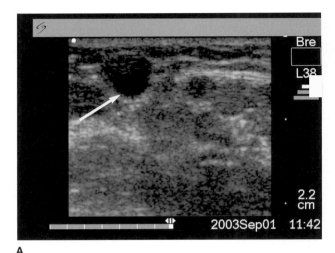

A

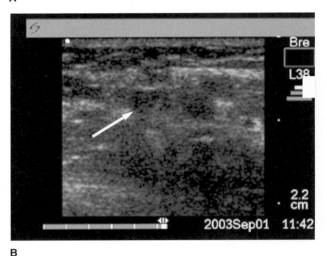

B

Figure 12.17   **(A)** Basilic vein (arrow). **(B)** Basilic vein compressed by transducer pressure (arrow).

Ultrasound imaging

Veins should be distended with the use of a tourniquet or sphygmomanometer prior to imaging for venous access. Imaging is best achieved in the transverse plane and should commence at a level just proximal to the elbow joint on the medial side of the limb with the arm in the anatomical position.

Vein identification and optimising visualisation

Using the positioning described above the operator should be able to identify the basilic vein. It is usually a solitary vessel and is easily compressible with pressure from the transducer (Figure 12.17). Moving the transducer slightly laterally allows visualisation of the brachial vein(s) and the accompanying artery. As with other sites the brachial vein is easily compressible but the artery is not. Also often the operator can clearly see the pulsatility of the arterial walls, which also helps to distinguish artery from vein. Moving the transducer more laterally usually reveals the cephalic vein as a solitary vein on the lateral side of the arm.

Positioning patient and equipment

The procedure is best performed with the patient in the supine position and the arm abducted to 45 degrees. The arm should be in the anatomical position. The operator should stand at the patient's side between the trunk and the abducted limb facing the patient's upper body. The US monitor should be placed facing the operator usually level with the patient's upper arm so that there is minimal effort for the operator to change glance between the puncture site and the US monitor.

US-guided upper limb venous puncture

Full aseptic technique must be used. Patient and operator positioning is described above. Vein selection depends on a number of factors including venous anatomy and anatomic variants, venous patency or thrombosis, and operator preferences. The authors prefer the basilic vein, other factors being equal, with a brachial puncture the second choice for venous access site. However in reality any of the named veins described above can be used for PICC insertion as can any other moderate-size vein identified in the upper limb.

Summary

Central venous catheters are placed by many operators and for numerous indications and the number of annual placements in the UK is estimated to be in the order of 200 000. Traditionally central venous access was achieved by blind needle puncture, the operator relying on anticipated patient anatomy to ensure correct venous access and the avoidance of inadvertent iatrogenic injury. The use of 2-D B-Mode ultrasound provides the operator with a simple and safe imaging technique that when correctly used will reduce the failure rate for venous access and reduce the incidence of procedural injury. Initial scanning prior to puncture will provide useful information regarding the proposed target vein including confirming its patency and suitability for CVC insertion, as well as demonstrating any aberrant vessels or other structures which may lie in the proposed needle path between skin and target vessel. The use of a sterile transducer cover and US gel permits the operator visualisation of the actual needle in real-time imaging throughout the entire length of its path from skin to target vessel thereby reducing the chance of procedural failure or incorrect vessel puncture. Finally after venous access has been achieved and a guidewire has been passed into the vessel US can be used to confirm that the wire is truly luminal within the target vessel. The skills required to use US for venous access require a knowledge of US anatomy of the vessels commonly used for CVC placement and the development of an appreciation of needle guidance based on 2-D US imaging. The necessary knowledge can easily be learned and the learning curve to achieve a satisfactory level of competence is relatively short. Therefore the technique of US needle guidance is likely to become the accepted standard for CVC placement.

13 Procedural applications of emergency bedside ultrasound

ANTHONY J DEAN, DANIEL K VINING

Objectives
The utility of ultrasound in the following common clinical problems and procedures is described:

- Foreign body localisation and removal
- Evaluation and management of soft tissue inflammatory conditions including cellulitis, abscess, haematoma, osteomyelitis
- Identification, localisation, and drainage of pleural fluid, ascites, and the urinary bladder
- Guidance in pericardiocentesis and pacemaker placement

Introduction

To the extent that phlebotomy, laryngoscopy and sigmoidoscopy are considered to be procedures, so too is ultrasound, performed at the bedside, by the treating physician. In contrast to the use of ultrasound as a diagnostic procedure, this chapter will focus on non-sonographic procedures that are guided or assisted by sonography. Occasionally, it may seem that more attention is being paid to diagnostic sonographic considerations than to procedural ones. Such attention is warranted because some relatively simple sonographic procedures require the underpinning of a relatively complex cognitive framework. For example, draining a bursa is simple; being certain that it is not a cellulitis, abscess, or septic joint is much more challenging, and no less important. The use of ultrasound in vascular access is treated in a separate chapter.

The reader of this chapter may get the occasional sense of *déjà vu* born of the fact that several techniques are shared by many procedural applications. Conversely, specific recommendations about technique are often vague, because they need to be determined by idiosyncratic factors that vary from case to case. Most gallstones and first trimester intrauterine pregnancies are alike; most abscesses and foreign bodies are not. In order to maximise the utility of ultrasound in a specific case, it is necessary to "think out of the box". A creative approach combined with a grasp of ultrasound physics, practice in its application, and familiarity with the strengths and limitations of available equipment, has the best chance of success.

Ultrasound in the evaluation and management of possible foreign bodies

Background

Wounds containing foreign bodies are at increased risk of delayed healing, prolonged inflammation, and infection.[1] Accurate identification and management of soft-tissue foreign bodies can be difficult for a variety of reasons. Lacerations and puncture wounds are sudden and unanticipated events, so that patients usually cannot give a definite history with respect to the presence or even likelihood of a foreign body. Physical examination is also often unreliable, especially in children and adults with an altered sensorium. In one retrospective series of 200 retained foreign bodies, it was determined that 38% of patients had been evaluated by a physician who had missed the diagnosis.[2] Missed foreign bodies in lacerations have been reported as a leading cause of medical malpractice lawsuits brought against emergency physicians in the United States.[3] Conversely, unnecessary exploration for a foreign body creates an iatrogenic wound, frequently in functionally important areas, which can lead to tissue damage, blood loss, and an increased risk of infection.

Although radiopaque foreign bodies (for example metal, glass, gravel) are usually easily seen on plain radiography, radiolucent objects such as wood and plastic are not. Ultrasonography has been used to identify nonradiopaque soft-tissue foreign bodies with variable success. Ultrasound also has the potential, in a clinical setting where access to fluoroscopy is limited, for precise real-time three-dimensional localisation of radiopaque foreign bodies. Sonographic localisation facilitates foreign body removal with smaller incisions and decreased dissection and operating time. Studies of this topic have been done *in vivo* and *in vitro*; the latter have involved both cadaver and animal tissue models.[4–10] Reported sensitivities have ranged from as high as 100%,[5,7] to as low as 50%, with only 70% specificity.[7] Most investigations find that ultrasonography with high frequency transducers, both *in* and *ex vivo*, is consistently accurate.[6,9–11]

The wide range of accuracies reported for sonographic identification of foreign bodies is due to several factors.

- First, the most common sites for foreign bodies are the extremities, especially the soles and palms. In these areas, multiple fascial planes can both mimic and obscure foreign bodies, and there can be technical difficulties in scanning small structures, such as fingers, and inaccessible areas, such as web spaces. Studies using models that do not reproduce these conditions tend to report higher accuracy.
- Second, smaller foreign bodies are harder to identify (by any technique) than large ones. One well controlled study showed almost 100% sensitivity for detecting 2–5 mm objects in the hand.[10] Certain foreign bodies – those smaller than the resolving power of a machine – will always be missed. Problems arising due to this purely technical limitation will diminish with increasing quality and affordability of bedside ultrasound equipment.
- Third, ultrasound is an operator dependent modality, and increasing experience is likely to be reflected by improved accuracy.[8]

In view of these issues, it would be prudent to discharge patients who appear to be free of foreign body after clinical evaluation (with or without ultrasound, radiographs, or foreign body removal) with clear warnings about the possibility of retained foreign body, and the need to return immediately should symptoms occur.

Technique and sonographic findings

In most circumstances, a higher frequency (6–12 MHz) linear array probe is preferred. This type of probe can image very superficial structures, and also, due to the parallel configuration of its beam, does not lose resolution at increasing depths. With the limited resources available in many emergency settings, a linear array probe may not be available. In this case, the use of an endocavitary probe, with higher frequencies and shorter focal length than a general-purpose abdominal transducer, has been described. Occasionally, especially when scanning bony or inaccessible areas such as the knuckles and web-spaces of the fingers and toes, a small footprint curved array probe is needed.

The skin should be cleansed, and the wound lavaged in the customary fashion. If the presence of a foreign body has already been ascertained with certainty based on clinical evaluation, and ultrasound is being used to provide additional structural or anatomic information, or if the patient is likely to be unable to tolerate the discomfort of the ultrasound examination, the area should be anaesthetised. The ultrasound probe needs to be covered by a sterile barrier. Dedicated covers for this purpose are available, but a sterile glove can be used. Since the powder in gloves is not sonolucent, it creates artefact and obscures the image, so that a "non-talc" glove should be utilised. Regular ultrasound gel can be placed inside the glove, but on the outside, sterile gel should be used. Pre-packaged sterile sachets are commercially available, but these dedicated products are not routinely stocked in many emergency departments (EDs). In that situation, sterile lubricating gel is easily accessible in most urethral catheterisation trays, and is an effective substitute.

The probe is placed on the skin and the area is systematically and slowly scanned through all tissue planes. As usual in emergency bedside ultrasound (EMBU), the power of ultrasound in the hands of the treating physician is in real-time scanning. Patients can often localise the foreign body with the symptoms caused by probe pressure. The location of deeply embedded foreign bodies may be sensed by patients even after the area has been locally anaesthetised. The entire area should be scanned in at least two orthogonal planes. The echoes generated by foreign bodies are highly dependent on the angle of the incident beam, with the best signals being generated when it is perpendicular to the long axis of the foreign body. It is therefore essential to scan in each direction, holding the probe face at a variety of angles to the skin surface. In addition to a hyperechoic focus, a variety of sonographic patterns has been described.[12,14] Wood almost always produces shadowing (Figure 13.1). Glass reliably causes reverberation artefact. Metallic foreign bodies may show either. Since the echo

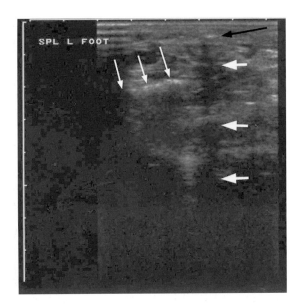

Figure 13.1   A wooden splinter which broke into two fragments in the foot. The first fragment crosses the plane of the ultrasound beam, but creates an echo (tip of black arrow) indistinguishable from surrounding soft tissue. Its presence is confirmed by the intense shadowing it causes (large white arrows). The second fragment is in the plane of the ultrasound beam, causing a linear echogenic focus (long white arrows). The shadowing caused by this foreign body is less pronounced, due to its width being less than that of the ultrasound beam.

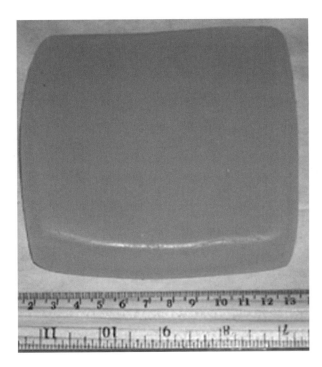

Figure 13.2   A commercially available spacer.

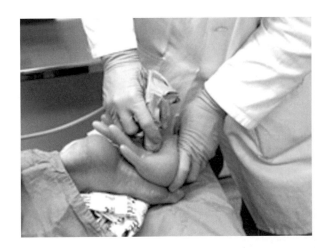

Figure 13.3   Use of a fluid filled glove for a spacer. The transducer is covered with a sterile glove.

may be indistinguishable from surrounding soft tissue, particular attention must be paid to evidence of unexplained shadowing. Chronic retained foreign bodies are often surrounded by a hypo-echoic halo of oedema or suppuration. Most foreign bodies are less than 1·6 cm below the surface.

Especially with puncture wounds caused by wood, the clinician may have a sense, based on mechanism and physical findings, of the likely orientation of the foreign body. This information is useful because it suggests the location and orientation of the echo pattern likely to be created by the foreign body, and to distinguish these from echoes created by dermal connective tissue. It also suggests angles to position the probe to maximise the strength of reflected echoes. The more sophisticated the ultrasound transducer, the narrower the thickness of the ultrasound beam ("beam width"). If the beam width exceeds the thickness of the foreign body, it may be impossible to identify the object when its long axis is parallel to the scanning plane. Thus, with the less technologically advanced equipment available in many emergency settings, foreign bodies may only

be identifiable when they are perpendicular to the scanning plane (see Figure 13.1).

If a foreign body is identified, care must be taken not to overlook a second or third. Wood and glass foreign bodies are especially prone to break in the soft tissues. To avoid this mistake, a complete scan should be completed after the identification of a foreign body and after its removal. Real-time scanning, as always, should be systematic and methodical, but needs to be done even more slowly than usual to avoid missing small objects.

Occasionally a superficial foreign body may be at a depth that is within the "near zone" of the ultrasound probe, preventing its visualisation. Most modern ultrasound probes are capable of resolving even the most superficial structures, but if it occurs, it can be overcome by the use of a "spacer" or "stand-off". These are sonolucent objects placed between the probe and the skin surface. They can also be used to allow a large object close to the skin to be seen within the angle of view subtended by a small footprint, curved array transducer. Spacers are commercially available, but are rarely maintained in the ED, and are cumbersome when needed for use in potentially contaminated areas, or for sterile procedures (see Figure 13.2). They can be effectively fashioned using a water filled examination glove (see Figure 13.3). Care must be taken to remove air and talc from the glove. Another technique is to completely immerse the area of interest in a water bath (see Figures 13.4A, B, C). This approach is particularly useful in the hand which can easily be manipulated in a water bath, and which may be especially difficult to image using routine methods, due to its angles, recesses, and thin dermis.

Once a foreign body is identified, it is necessary to modify customary sonographic scanning technique. Attention to the screen becomes secondary to detailed scrutiny of the wound site, landmarks on the skin, and the location of the

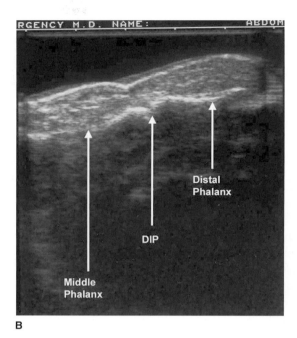

B

Figure 13.4(B) Longitudinal view of digit in water bath, demonstrating an excellent view of the soft tissues (no foreign body is present). The cortices of the phalanges are easily seen, as is the distal interphalangeal joint (DIP). The flexor digitorum profundus tendon can also be seen.

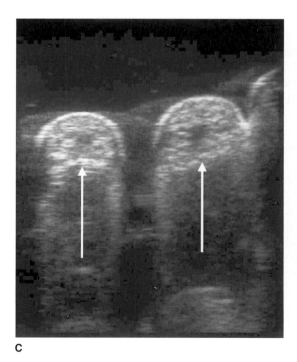

C

Figure 13.4(C) Transverse view of the fingers in a water bath. The cortices of the phalanges (arrows) cause shadowing. Above them on the image the flexor tendons can be seen as dark areas.

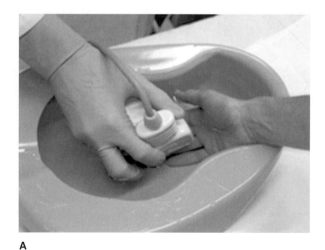

A

Figure 13.4(A) Technique for scanning using a water bath.

transducer. Similarly to the technique used in vascular access, the object is placed under the centre of the probe. With the probe at right angles to the skin surface, the callipers should be utilised to ascertain its depth and transverse dimensions in real time. Repetitive real-time scanning through the object will allow three-dimensional conceptualisation of the foreign body and its position relative to other structures, especially tendons and fascial planes. If necessary, marker points can be placed on the skin with overlying echogenic pellets to correlate marks and sonographic findings. Since sterile indelible pens are usually not available, the imprint made by pressing an object onto the skin for 10–20 seconds (for example the hub of a syringe) will hold for the time needed to remove the foreign body.

For larger or longer objects, a single operator can identify, localise, and remove most foreign bodies. A single operator may wish to hold the transducer in one hand and introduce a haemostat or forcep with the other, and remove the foreign body with direct real-time sonographic visualisation. Another technique is to introduce needles that can be passed under direct sonographic visualisation to the foreign body. It has been demonstrated that the best technique is to use two needles in the same plane, but perpendicular to one another, that meet immediately below the foreign body. The needles are left in place, and the transducer is removed from the field. An incision is made down one of the needles to the foreign body, with the second one allowing for an identification of the depth at which the object will be found. If small or friable foreign bodies are identified, it may be necessary to use a "two person" technique. After the skin is anaesthetised, the first member of the team obtains real-time images of the foreign body while the surgical operator dedicates both hands to the task of locating and removing it. As with any attempt at foreign body removal, careful preparatory measures to ensure a bloodless field are well worth the little extra effort, and are more likely to be rewarded with success.

Caveats and potential pitfalls

Multiple tissue planes, scar tissue, and air in a laceration may both obscure a foreign body or give the appearance of one, when none is there. Fresh haematoma may have the same echodensity as the foreign body, thus obscuring its presence. Normal structures such as sesamoid bones,

ossification centres, calcified cartilage, or other soft tissue calcifications may be mistaken for foreign bodies. Small radiopaque foreign bodies are easily identified on radiographs, but may be missed on ultrasound. Ultrasound should not be used absolutely to rule out soft tissue foreign bodies, especially when there is a high index of clinical suspicion.

Pearls and pitfalls: foreign body localisation

Subcutaneous tissues, especially in the palms and soles

- can be mistaken for foreign bodies
- can obscure foreign bodies

Multiple foreign bodies

- especially with splinter and glass injuries
- complete, systematic, real-time scanning after localisation of first foreign body
- re-scan after removal of foreign body

Difficult to access areas

- consider the use of a small footprint probe
- consider the use of a "stand off"
- consider the use of a water bath

Foreign body removal

- consider local anatomic structures
- identify local structures sonographically where possible
- consider structural integrity of foreign body in choosing a technique for removal

The "negative" exam

- be cautious about telling patients that foreign body has been definitively excluded
- counsel patients about symptoms of retained foreign body after a "negative" sonographic evaluation, or an apparently successful removal

---

Ultrasound evaluation of cellulitis, abscess, and other soft tissue inflammatory conditions

Background

The differential diagnosis in patients presenting with symptoms of soft tissue inflammation – *rubor, tumor, calor and dolor* – includes cellulitis, abscess, phlebitis, neoplasm, pyomyositis, fasciitis, haematoma, lymphadenopathy, tendonitis, bursitis, and joint effusions. While clinical information may be helpful, it is rarely sufficient for a definite diagnosis, and often only serves to break this list into groups based on anatomic location. Soft tissue inflammation in the trunk and extremities is usually due to either abscess or cellulitis. These are indistinguishable in the absence of pointing or frankly draining pus. Occasionally, the same clinical picture signals the presence of more malignant processes such as pyomyositis, osteomyelitis, or necrotising fasciitis. In the hands and feet, unrecognised abscess is less likely, but cellulitis can be confused with tendonitis and occult foreign body. Pain and swelling in the vicinity of a joint may be due to an inflammatory process within the joint, usually mandating arthrocentesis, or to overlying bursitis and cellulitis, both of which would strongly contraindicate arthrocentesis in view of the potential for iatrogenic septic arthritis. In most joints, including the hip, shoulder, wrist, elbow, and ankle, this distinction is difficult on clinical grounds alone (Figure 13.5). Swelling and tenderness accompany healing post-operative surgical wounds, but also may be due to soft tissue infection, haematomata, and abscesses. Haematomata may also develop atraumatically in patients on anticoagulants. In the inguinal area, tender swollen lymphadenopathy and femoral artery aneurysms are potential aetiologies. Masses in the popliteal space may be due to Baker cysts and aneurysms. Bedside ultrasound has the capacity either to diagnose these conditions (for example abscess versus cellulitis), or to permit further diagnostic testing that will lead to their identification (for example joint effusion versus bursitis versus cellulitis).[12] In addition, ultrasound can be of assistance in the execution of subsequent procedures, where indicated (for example needle aspiration and/or incision and drainage).

Technique and sonographic findings

The choice of transducer is based on similar considerations to those discussed in the section on foreign bodies. A high frequency (5–10 MHz) linear array probe is usually ideal, although a convex general purpose probe or endocavitary probe may allow better surface contact in certain locations such as the oropharynx, or in the web spaces of the hand or foot. Liberal amounts of conducting gel should be applied to the area in question and the probe slowly swept over it, starting in an area of normal tissue, then the area of interest, and continuing until tissue is normal again. Views

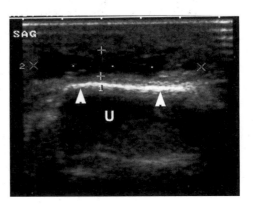

Figure 13.5 This patient presented with pain, erythema, and swelling of the posterior aspect of the proximal forearm and elbow. Olecranon bursitis was suspected, despite the unusually wide area of surrounding cellulitis. Ultrasound demonstrated a fluid collection with highly irregular margins suggestive of an abscess (between callipers), overlying the proximal ulna (U, cortex indicated by arrowheads). It was tapped using ultrasound guidance (see Figures 13.14B and 13.16).

should be obtained in at least two orthogonal planes, allowing the sonographer to develop a three-dimensional conceptual image of the area of interest. Sonographic and clinical findings should be correlated, noting sites where symptoms are elicited with probe pressure. Scanning should be slow and methodical to avoid missing subtle variations of echogenicity or small sonolucent areas, both of which can represent pockets of pus.

Acoustic standoffs, either commercial or fabricated out of an examination glove filled with water and carefully de-aired, may be employed to visualise superficial areas of interest, allowing them to be placed within the probe's focal zone (see Figures 13.2 and 13.3).[13] Both cellulitis and abscess can be extremely tender, so that the lightest probe pressure consistent with a good acoustical interface should be maintained. Occasionally local anaesthetic or systemic sedation is needed. If areas with broken skin need to be scanned, the probe should be placed inside a sterile protective sheath as explained in the section on foreign bodies. Sonographic techniques and findings for specific soft tissue inflammatory conditions are as follows.

Cellulitis

Ultrasonography of cellulitis usually reveals thickening of the skin and underlying tissue (see

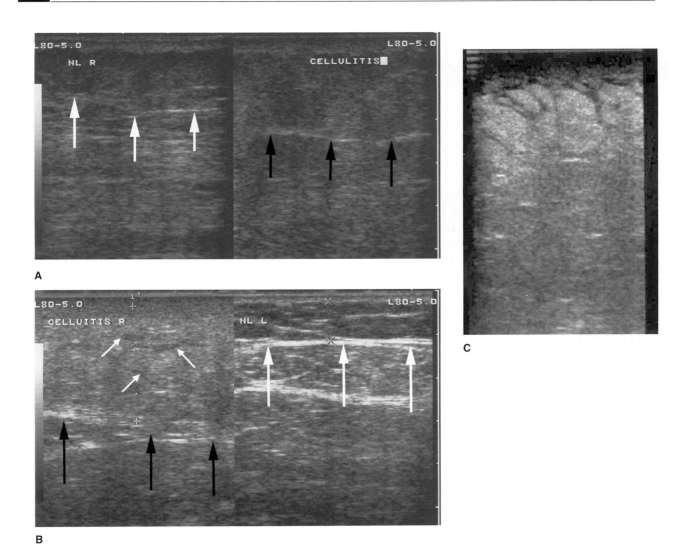

Figure 13.6 Various sonographic appearances of cellulitis. **(A)** Comparison of normal with cellulitic subcutaneous tissue of the abdominal wall. On the left hand side of the image, the thickness of the subcutaneous fat is revealed by the depth of the subdermal fascia (white arrows). On the contralateral side, in the area of symptoms, the dermis is thicker (black arrows), and much more echogenic. **(B)** Cellulitis of the thigh. In this case, the normal subcutaneous tissue is shown on the right of the image, and is 8·9 mm thick (white arrows showing superficial fascia). On the left of the image, the dermis is 26·5 mm thick, more echogenic, with traces of interlobular oedema (small white arrows). The superficial fascia is also thickened from oedema (black arrows). **(C)** Thick reticular bands of oedema surrounding lobules of cellulitic adipose tissue. The patient was extremely obese with thick pannus, which is diffusely hyperechoic and obscures the superficial muscle fascia.

Figures 13.6A,B,C). Thickening can be identified objectively by using the electronic callipers to measure the distance from the skin surface to the superficial fascia in the area of interest, and comparing it to a contralateral area of normal skin. Cellulitic tissue is usually hyperechoic, although occasionally it is hypo-echoic. The hyperechoic fat lobules have a cobblestone appearance; between them there appear lacy anechoic bands in a reticular pattern, usually ascribed to thickened oedematous interlobular septa.[12] At the margins of cellulitis, the transition from normal to abnormal is gradual. Telltale foci of soft tissue gas include punctate hyperechoic foci sometimes with shimmering reverberation artefact (see Figure 13.7D).

At the conclusion of a sonographic examination, if a patient's soft tissue inflammation appears to be due to cellulitis, not abscess, careful consideration should be given to the possibility of a deeper infection such as pyomyositis or fasciitis (see below). Cellulitis and soft tissue oedema may have similar ultrasonographic appearances, but can usually be distinguished clinically. In contrast to lymphoedema, which typically appears as diffuse swelling of the subcutaneous fat and muscle, the swelling of cellulitis remains confined to the subcutaneous fat.

Abscess

Abscesses may develop *de novo*, as the result of penetrating trauma, or as suppurative sequellae to cellulitis. Due to the fact that their formation and development are dynamic, a variety of sonographic appearances have been described (Figure 13.7A). Most commonly a hypo-echoic cavity surrounded by a relatively hyperechoic rim, reflecting a "mature" abscess, is seen (Figures 13.7A and 13.7B). Colour flow Doppler analysis of the abscess will reveal the hyperechoic rim to be hypervascular, and absence of flow within the abscess. Posterior acoustic enhancement is common (Figure 13.7A). The margins are often irregular with or without septations, correlating with the clinical finding of loculations that need to be broken down when an abscess is drained (Figures 13.7B and 13.7C). Heterogeneous internal echoes may also be seen due to debris within the abscess cavity (Figures 13.7B and 13.7C). In scanning at sites of injection drug abuse, the sonographer should look for evidence of foreign bodies that have both therapeutic and practical consequences for the physician performing the drainage procedure. Echoes within the abscess cavity, often mobile, nondependent, with a glistening appearance, and with posterior ring-down

artefact, may be caused by gas forming organisms in the abscess (see Figure 13.7D). As noted for cellulitis, sparkling echoes with posterior reverberation artefact arising in the soft tissues suggest a more dangerous necrotising soft tissue infection. Abscesses generally displace and do not cross fascial planes. Rarely an abscess erodes into a fascial plane, leading to an elongated spindle-shaped hypo-echoic shape, making it difficult to distinguish from non-inflammatory fluid collections such as post-operative haematomata and seromata or ruptured Baker cysts.

Less commonly, but more problematically, abscesses may also be hyperechoic or iso-echoic. The former must be distinguished from solid tumours and nodes, and the latter can easily be overlooked completely. Several techniques have been described to overcome this potential blind spot in the sonographic evaluation of the soft tissues. Subtle differences between the echogenicity of an abscess and the surrounding tissues may be accentuated by scanning at several frequencies, varying the dynamic range and gain settings. If the ultrasound machine has tissue harmonic capability, the area should be scanned using both modes. Power Doppler assessment may also help to resolve the issue, showing, as noted above, a rim of increased flow with an avascular core. Even hyperechoic abscesses may cause posterior acoustical enhancement, so the deeper tissues should be checked for this finding (Figure 13.7E). Finally, ambiguities might be clarified with dynamic assessment using local digital and/or

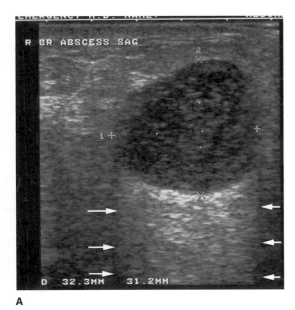

A

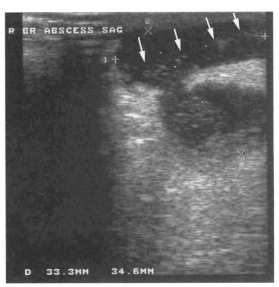

B

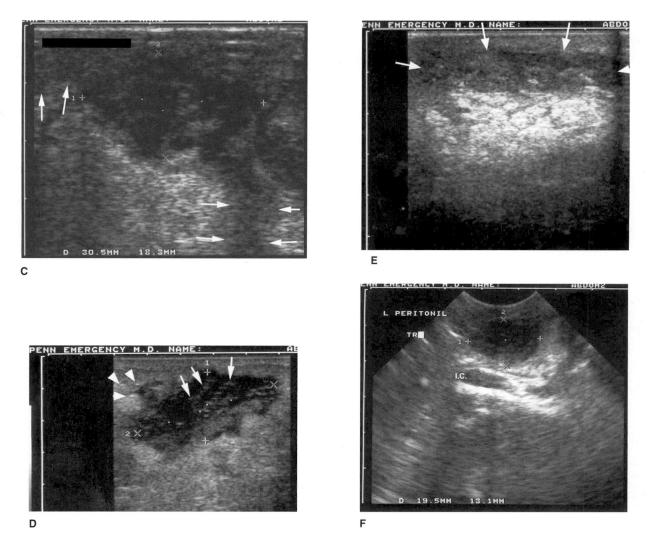

Figure 13.7 Various sonographic appearances of abscesses. **(A)** A breast abscess with hyperechoic surrounding soft tissue. In this view it appears unilocular with regular walls, although in other views, the abscess was shown to have extensive and complex loculations (see Figure 13.7B). Note the posterior acoustical enhancement caused by the abscess cavity (the apparent band of hyperechoic tissue between the arrows). **(B)** Another section of the abscess in Figure 13.7(A) showing irregular loculations connected by thin fistulous tracts. Note the irregular internal echodensities with a fluid-fluid level caused by the layering of pus and sediment within the abscess (arrows). **(C)** An abscess with irregular borders and heterogeneous internal debris. Some of the surrounding tissues are hypo-echoic (arrows), suggesting ongoing suppuration. **(D)** An abscess with irregular margins at the site of injection drug abuse. Floating streams of shimmering echogenic foci, better appreciated in real time, indicated gas (arrows), which was also seen in the surrounding soft tissues (arrowheads). Reverberation artefact, often seen with gas, is not seen in this example. **(E)** An iso-echoic abscess. This abscess (arrows) might easily be mistaken for cellulitis if the strong posterior acoustical enhancement (see Figure 13.7A) is overlooked. **(F)** A peritonsillar abscess (callipers). Note the close proximity of the internal carotid artery (IC).

probe pressure. If an abscess is present, pressure applied digitally adjacent to the transducer, alternating with direct probe pressure, may show a characteristic "to and fro" pattern of the fluid collection in the tissues. Clearly, in the absence of liquefaction, tissues will compress uniformly, and there will be no appearance of flow. In the case of hyperechoic abscess, the same technique can be used to distinguish it from a solid soft tissue tumour.

If an abscess is identified, its extent and approximate size should be assessed. The optimal site for incision and drainage should be determined, usually based on the site where the abscess is most superficial. The location of contiguous neurovascular structures should be noted, where applicable (for example in the groin or axilla). The probe is centred over the point of the abscess and indelible marks are placed at both ends of the probe in perpendicular orientations, creating two intersecting lines for incision. Due to cosmetic or anatomic considerations, needle aspiration may be preferable to incision in certain locations, such as the head, neck, or breast. The method for ultrasound guided needle aspiration is explained in detail in the section on drainage of joints and bursae.

Peritonsillar abscess

In ambulatory medicine, a common diagnostic dilemma in patients presenting with sore throat is that between peritonsillar cellulitis ("peritonsillitis", treated with antibiotics) and peritonsillar abscess ("quinsy", treated with surgical drainage). Clinical evaluation alone is unreliable, and use of needle aspiration for diagnosis is problematic for several reasons. First it, too, is unreliable; second it is potentially dangerous in view of the close proximity of the carotid artery; and third, it is distressing and painful for the patient. Computed tomography of the neck is an alternative, but is not universally available, has associated logistical and temporal delays, is more expensive, and requires the use of intravenous contrast agents and ionising radiation. Studies of ultrasound for this purpose have shown a sensitivity of about 90%, and specificity of 83–100%. An endocavitary probe with a protective sheath is used (Figure 13.8). Topical anaesthetic may be applied to the tonsillar area, but is not needed for most patients. Most abscesses appear as hypoechoic collections, but, similar to findings for cutaneous abscesses, a minority is iso-echoic (Figure 13.7F). Therefore, if an abscess is not identified, the tonsil (a discrete iso-echoic mass) should be sonographically located. Any other mass, regardless of echopattern, probably represents abscess, which is usually found immediately adjacent to the tonsil.

If an abscess is identified, needle aspiration has been shown to be equally effective, simpler, and less invasive than incision and drainage. A sonographic determination is made of the size and depth of the abscess, the optimal site for needle aspiration, and the location of the carotid artery. The anxiety experienced by the clinician performing blind needle drainage of quinsy is supported by a study that found that

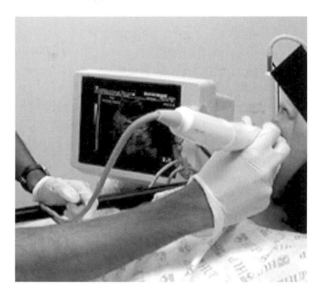

Figure 13.8 Technique for use of an endocavitary probe to diagnose peritonsillar abscess.

the average distance from the mucosal surface to the abscess is a full 9 mm, while the distance from the abscess to the carotid artery can be as little as 4 mm.

Needle aspiration with direct, real-time ultrasound guidance has been reported, but is often impracticable without a dedicated probe-mounted needle guide, due to the confined space and patient discomfort. If it is attempted without a needle guide, a long needle (for example 10 cm spinal needle) should be used. Usually it is easier, first to locate sonographically the optimal site for needle aspiration, and subsequently, with unimpeded visual access and two hands free, to perform the procedure.

Fasciitis and pyomyositis

Necrotising fasciitis may occur as a sequella to trauma, but often arises spontaneously in immune-compromised patients, especially those with diabetes. Pyomyositis used to be considered rare outside of the tropics, but it also is seen in patients with impaired immunity. With a normal or nonspecific sonographic evaluation of soft tissue inflammation, a high clinical index of suspicion needs to be maintained for these diseases, due to their nonspecific clinical findings and their fulminant course if untreated. Sonographic evaluation during their early treatable phase may reveal oedema, fascial thickening, or subtle abnormalities of echogenicity, but ultrasound cannot reliably exclude these diseases. With progression of disease, hypo-echoic bands of pus develop along the fascial planes, with persistent thickening of the dermis. As noted in the discussion of cellulitis, sonographic evidence of gas should be sought: sparkling intensely hyperechoic foci with shimmering posterior reverberation artefact. Infected muscle may not show sonographic changes until the onset of frank liquefaction.

Haematoma

Haematoma may occur within the fascial planes, subcutaneous tissues, or intramuscularly. Intramuscular haematoma may be iso-echoic with muscle if it contains freshly clotted blood, so careful examination for interruption of the usual ordered striations of muscle should be sought (Figure 13.9A and 13.9B). The techniques described above for the distinction of iso-echoic abscess from cellulitis should be used. In addition to good technique, high-resolution equipment may help. Subdermal and intermuscular haematomata dissect along tissue planes creating elongated flattened areas of sonolucency. Compared with abscesses they tend to be less tender and more extensive. Evaluation of the surrounding tissues with grey scale and power Doppler is less likely to reveal the hyperechoic and hypervascular pattern typically seen with an abscess.

Lymph nodes and other nodular masses

Lymph nodes frequently cause tender inflammatory masses in the axilla, groin, and elsewhere. Unlike abscesses, they tend to have smooth margins, without a hyperechoic surrounding rim (Figures 13.10A and 13.10B). They classically demonstrate internal echoes, but these, in contrast to those of abscess or haematoma with clot, are well organised. Usually the cortex of the node is relatively hypo-echoic, with the medulla relatively hyperechoic. As usual, systematic real-time scanning is mandatory, since it can identify the typical configuration of nodes: they are multiple and discrete. A variety of non-acute causes of soft tissue swelling can also be identified sonographically, and should be differentiated from lymph nodes. These include lipomata (well marginated, compressible, with diffuse heterogeneous inner echoes), and rheumatoid, sarcoid, or tophaceous nodules. These are usually identifiable to the examining physician, based on the clinical context.

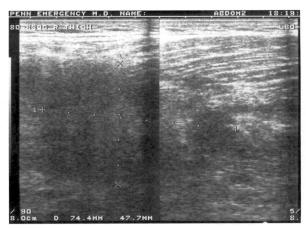

A

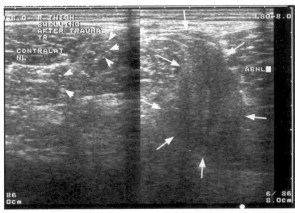

B

Figure 13.9 A patient presenting with two hours' progressive posterior thigh pain after forceful hip extension. **(A)** In the sagittal view the ordered longitudinal striations of the muscle can be seen to be interrupted by the diffusely, mildly heterogeneous echodensity of the haematoma (callipers). **(B)** On the right hand side, the same haematoma is seen in transverse view (arrows). On the left, a view of the normal contralateral thigh is shown, the striations of which appear as punctate echodensities (arrowheads). The longitudinal extent can be appreciated in real time.

Osteomyelitis

The utility of plain radiographs in the diagnosis of this disease is limited due to the several weeks' delay prior to radiographically identifiable bony changes, and the frequent occurrence of this disease at old fracture sites, making radiographic interpretation difficult. Ultrasound is also limited in its ability to identify osteomyelitis due to its inability to penetrate cortical bone. However, several sonographic abnormalities have been described, including joint effusions, peri-osteal swelling, and sub- and supra-periosteal fluid

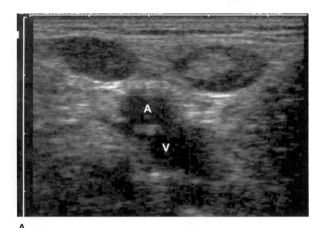

A

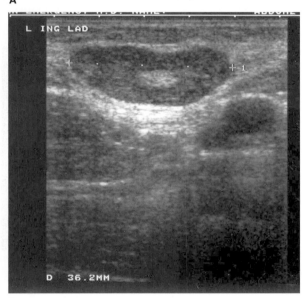

B

Figure 13.10 Lymph nodes. Note the normal echodensity of surrounding soft tissue, and the smooth margins, arguing against an acute inflammatory process. The lack of acoustic drop off in lymph nodes may cause posterior enhancement, and does not necessarily indicate suppuration. **(A)** Two lymph nodes overlying the common femoral artery (A) and vein (V). **(B)** A large lymph node (callipers, note dimensions), with characteristic hyperechoic medulla.

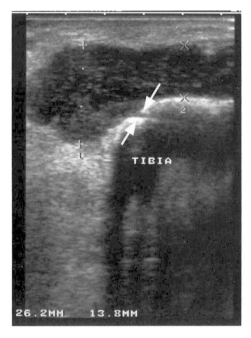

Figure 13.11 Osteomyelitis at the site of a gunshot wound from approximately 10 years earlier. The presence of internal fixation devices made interpretation of plain films difficult. The peri-osteal abscess with internal echoes can be seen (callipers); as well as the sinus tract through the tibial cortex (arrows).

collections (see Figure 13.11).[17] The most sensitive and specific finding is a fluid collection directly adjacent to cortical bone. Strikingly, peri-osteal fluid collections are found in many patients with osteomyelitis who have less than four days of symptoms. In sickle cell patients this finding is less specific since it can also represent bone infarct in vaso-occlusive crisis. However, even in this group, the distinction can usually be made due to the fact that in the latter condition the peri-osteal fluid collection is almost always

< 10 mm in thickness, whereas in osteomyelitis it is 10 mm or greater. If the issue is still in doubt, it can be easily resolved with ultrasound-guided aspiration of the fluid collection. At sites of prior fracture or chronic osteomyelitis, cortical defects may be identified. With adjacent peri-osteal fluid, these are almost pathognomonic for osteomyelitis. Needle aspiration of peri-osteal fluid collections is as described below for joints and bursae.

Needle drainage of joints, bursae, and tendons

As noted above, it is necessary to determine whether inflammatory symptoms in the region of joints are due to acute arthritis or overlying bursitis, tendonitis, or cellulitis (Figure 13.5). The location and sonographic identification of ligaments and tendons is dealt with elsewhere in this text. Once a distended joint or bursa is identified, needle aspiration is usually the next step. Typical anatomic locations for joint effusions and bursae are beyond the scope of the present discussion, and are well covered elsewhere. With most joints, the site of maximal soft tissue swelling and/or fluctuance can be

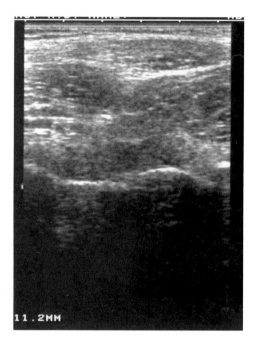

Figure 13.12 Sonogram of the left hip, showing effusion.

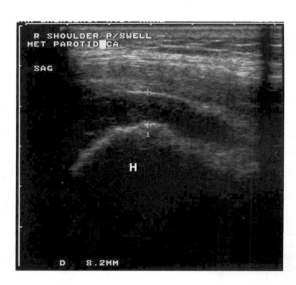

Figure 13.13 Longitudinal sonogram of the humeral head (H) in a patient with a tender swollen shoulder and thrombocytopenia due to metastatic cancer. A large effusion is present (between callipers) with internal echoes, which are consistent with either pus or clot in the joint, although pus often forms a layer. Note the irregular appearance of the bony cortex, which on further imaging was shown to be due to osteoarthritis, not metastatic disease.

identified by physical examination, which directs and focusses subsequent sonographic evaluation. Deep joints, particularly the hips and shoulders, are often not amenable to this approach. Hips are imaged with the ultrasound probe aligned along the femoral neck: usually at about 45 degrees to the cephalocaudal axis. Effusion causes the joint capsule to be deflected anteriorly, creating a hypo-echoic area anterior to the femoral neck (Figure 13.12). The primary area of examination is the "anterior recess", which is found immediately below the femoral head. Experts make contradictory claims as to the optimal hip position for augmentation of small effusions.[12,18–20] If the patient is able to move the hip, positioning should be arranged on an individual basis. The average thickness of the fluid stripe is less than 2·5 mm in adults and teenagers, and less than 4·5 mm in children less than 11 years old. A difference of greater than 2–3 mm compared to the asymptomatic side is considered significant, although in most acutely inflamed hips, the difference far exceeds this margin.[21] If no effusion is identified, the lateral thigh should be evaluated for bursitis. Arthrocentesis of the hip is performed lateral to the femoral sheath.

The shoulder is scanned with the probe axis bridging the joint space (the probe will be rotated as it moves from anterior to posterior). Effusions tend to cause the joint capsule to protrude anteriorly or posteriorly, but a systematic scan just distal to the acromion process from anterior to posterior will identify other structures around the joint, including the subacromial bursae, and the biceps and rotator cuff tendons, all of which are potential causes of a painful shoulder (Figure 13.13). If the patient places the hand on the opposite shoulder the fluid in the joint space on the posterior view can be augmented. If a shoulder effusion is identified, it is usually tapped, as described below, using this posterior approach.

If fluid is identified around any joint, its origin (for example synovial, peritendonous, bursal) should be determined, along with its size, location, and optimal access site, avoiding surrounding soft tissue structures. If the fluid is synovial in origin, the examiner should determine whether it can be augmented by manipulating the joint or surrounding tissues. With small joints (such as the wrist or ankle), this will facilitate access and the likelihood of obtaining adequate quantities of fluid. If the patient is unable to reproduce these manipulations, the examiner will need to enlist the help of an assistant to perform them while the arthrocentesis is performed.

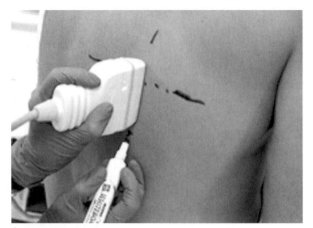

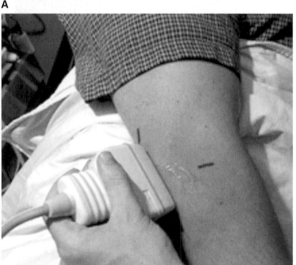

B

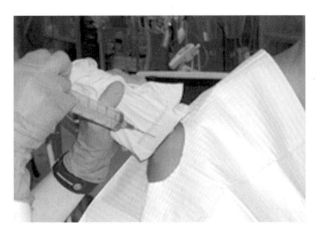

Figure 13.15   Arthrocentesis of the shoulder using the "one-step" approach, in which one hand is used for sonographic guidance, while the other simultaneously performs the procedure. The probe is placed inside a sterile glove. The plane of the transducer is at approximate right angles to the path of the needle. The depth of the effusion, and the anticipated path to it, are established prior to insertion of the needle.

Figure 13.14   The two-step approach to drainage procedures is preferred when large volumes are anticipated (requiring more time, for example pleural effusions or ascites, 13.14A) as well as for smaller, less accessible targets (for example ankle, elbow, or wrist effusions 13.14B). The skin is marked prior to prepping and draping the patient.
(A) Sonographic marking of a pleural effusion. The patient should be in a comfortable position and not move between the marking and the procedure. **(B)** Sonographic marking of abscess adjacent to the proximal ulna.

Ultrasound guidance in the aspiration can be performed using one of two techniques. The first, often preferable with small or superficial fluid collections (for example wrist or elbow effusions, olecranon bursa), or those in hard to access sites (for example ankle), uses a two-step approach. This is similar to that described above for peritonsillar abscess (Figures 13.14A and 13.14B). Preferably a high frequency (6–12 MHz) linear array probe is utilised. The optimal site for needle access is

sonographically identified and placed under the centre of the transducer. Indelible marks are placed on the skin at either end of the probe in two perpendicular directions, creating two intersecting lines over the site of needle aspiration. Prominent local bony landmarks are identified (for example the distal tibia and talus in the ankle, or distal radius and proximal carpus in the wrist), and their relationship with the targeted fluid collection. The ultrasound probe is then removed, and the skin prepped, draped, and tapped, using the previously identified and placed landmarks.

The second technique, similar to that used for vascular access and foreign body localisation, uses real-time sonography during the procedure (Figure 13.15). This technique is likely to be superior for deeper fluid collections, such as hip or shoulder effusions, where it may also be necessary to use a lower frequency (for example 5 MHz) probe. After careful cleansing of the skin, sonographic gel is liberally applied to the transducer, which is placed within a sterile protective sheath (or sterile unpowdered examination glove). A high frequency "small parts" probe is usually ideal, although in certain situations massive oedema or obesity may make it necessary to use a lower frequency probe, with better penetration. Sterile sonographic gel is placed on the outside of the sheath. The operator holds the transducer in the non-dominant hand with the syringe for aspiration in the other. The transducer is placed on the skin and used to confirm the location for easiest and most direct access to the joint or bursa. The probe is adjusted so that the sonographic image of the anticipated insertion site is centred on the screen, in order that the needle can subsequently be inserted precisely under the middle of the probe. The probe is then slid sufficiently away from this site to allow access of the needle, usually about 5–10 mm. The orientation of the probe on the skin surface is 90 degrees to the arthrocentesis needle. By rocking the transducer, it is possible to identify the needle soon after it has penetrated the skin. The needle may be seen as an echogenic focus with posterior shadowing, or, more frequently, only the shadowing is seen (Figure 13.16). For superficial effusions (such as those typically encountered in the wrist or the anterior approach to the ankle), the needle will enter the joint space almost immediately. In this situation, real-time ultrasound verifies complete evacuation of the joint fluid, and avoids the risk of trauma to the joint by attempts to remove fluid that is not there. With deeper effusions (such as those typically found in the shoulder), it provides guidance to the effusion, as well as real-time visual confirmation of evacuation. As noted above, an assistant may be needed to manipulate the joint or surrounding area to maximise the volume of accessible synovial fluid.

Ultrasound guidance in assessment of pleural fluid, ascites, and the urinary bladder

General remarks about technique for thoracentesis, paracentesis, and bladder aspiration

A transducer should be chosen which gives an adequate field of view with maximal resolution, but with adequate penetration to reach the far wall of the target fluid collection. As with the evaluation of soft tissue fluid collections, different probes offer advantages depending on the clinical situation. To obtain images through a small acoustic window (for example between the ribs, or of an infant's bladder), a small footprint or phased array probe will be advantageous. When space constraints are not an issue, or to view large fluid collections, a larger footprint probe is preferable.

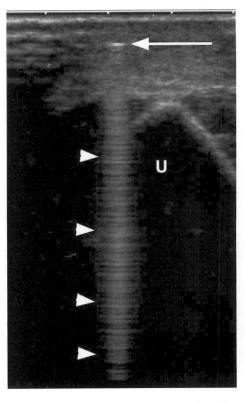

Figure 13.16 Reverberation artefact (arrowheads) caused by the needle (arrow) being advanced over the proximal ulna (U), draining the abscess described in Figures 13.5 and 13.14B.

As described for aspiration of joint fluid, ultrasound can be performed using either a two-step technique (localise the optimal site, mark the skin, prep and drape the patient, perform the procedure, see Figure 13.14A) or one-step method (ultrasound providing real-time images of the passage of the needle to the target, Figure 13.15). In general, the former, (two-step method) is adequate for larger targets (for example large collections of ascites, distended bladders in adults), whereas the latter, which is logistically slightly more cumbersome, may be preferred for smaller, less accessible targets (for example small pleural effusions, bladders in infants, localised pockets of ascites). If no fluid is aspirated, re-evaluation with ultrasound should be performed to assess for movement of the effusion or the need for a larger needle.

Thoracentesis

Thoracentesis is usually performed for either therapeutic evacuation of a large symptomatic fluid collection, or for the diagnosis of a pleural effusion. Ultrasound performed at the bedside by the treating clinician lends several advantages in this procedure. Ultrasound is more accurate in the localisation of small effusions than decubitus radiographs and when used to guide thoracentesis has a lower rate of serious complications than a blind approach. When the ultrasound is performed by the treating clinician at the bedside, delays, logistical impediments associated with patient transfer, as well as the risk of removal of the patient from the resuscitation area, are all avoided. Finally, for patients on ventilators, lateral decubitus radiographs are impracticable, and ultrasound is superior in differentiating pleural effusions from a lower lobe infiltrate, atelectasis, consolidation, or elevated hemi-diaphragm, than portable upright radiographs in these patients.

Procedure

As with blind thoracentesis, patients who are able to, usually undergo the procedure in the sitting position, although with sonographic guidance it can also be accomplished in the supine and lateral decubitus positions. In all cases, longitudinal scans are initiated in the most dependent area of the thorax. Fluid identified elsewhere represents a loculated effusion. Pleural fluid usually appears as a dependent anechoic collection with an echogenic border at its interface with aerated lung. This may often be seen to move within the effusion with respiration. Empyema or haemothorax may have internal echoes or septations (Figure 13.17).

The following features should be used to confirm that a hypo-echoic region on a sonogram is a pleural effusion:

- it is anatomic, not artefactual (for example from rib shadowing)
- it is superior to the diaphragm
- the near border is bounded by the straight echogenic line of the parietal pleura
- the far border is bounded by lung behind the effusion
- there is dynamic respiratory variation of the distance between the parietal and visceral pleura.

Scanning through the transverse, sagittal, and oblique planes around the site of the planned thoracentesis should be performed to evaluate for the presence of lung, heart, and diaphragm. Authorities recommend that for safe thoracentesis,

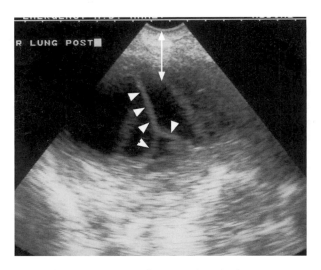

Figure 13.17 A pleural effusion with multiple septations (arrowheads). The abnormally irregular margins of the cavity, and its depth (double headed arrow) suggest pleural thickening, although it could possibly be due to adherent atelectatic lung. This would not be a good site to use for pleurocentesis.

the effusion be at least 15 mm in depth from the parietal to the visceral pleura throughout the respiratory cycle, with effusion also identified one rib space above and below.[22] Due to the difficulty of attaining real-time images through the intercostal space at the same time as introducing a needle, most authorities recommend the "two-step" method as described in "Technique", above. For this reason, the distance between the skin surface and the parietal pleura should be measured by ultrasound, so that the length of needle required, and the distance it will need to be inserted, are known prior to performing the procedure. The skin is marked, taking special care that mobile skin folds are not being displaced by the ultrasound probe. The patient must be kept absolutely still while the area is prepped and draped, and standard sterile thoracentesis is accomplished, usually within one minute.

Complications

In two large series of ultrasound-guided thoracentesis in a high-risk group of intensive care unit patients, complications occurred in less than 2·4%. The most common was pneumo-thorax, which occurred in about 1%.[22,23] Large studies of patients who are able to sit for the procedure have achieved pneumothorax rates of 0%, even accessing small loculated effusions.[24,25]

Numerous studies have examined the need for post-thoracentesis chest radiograph and have reported that it is not necessary in all cases. Risk factors for post-thoracentesis pneumothorax include mechanical ventilation, aspiration of air, prior thoracic irradiation, abnormal thoracic anatomy, multiple attempts, and symptoms of pneumothorax.[26] Post-procedure chest radiography may be safely confined to only those patients with risk factors. Other serious side effects include haemothorax, organ laceration, and re-expansion pulmonary oedema. Re-expansion pulmonary oedema, usually thought to occur following rapid re-expansion of a chronically collapsed lung, may also occur in lung that has only been collapsed a short time or in a gently re-expanded lung.

Paracentesis

The most common therapeutic indication for paracentesis is for the relief of tense ascites, which can cause intense discomfort and cardiovascular and respiratory compromise. In the emergency setting, the usual diagnostic indication is the identification of spontaneous bacterial peritonitis. Occasionally it is also indicated for the diagnosis of other causes of new or unexplained ascites, such as carcinomatosis.

In comparison to thoracentesis, descriptions of ultrasound-guidance in paracentesis are limited. This may be because the complications of blind paracentesis are rare and usually less serious than those of thoracentesis. It also may be that the presence of a moderate pleural effusion is more easily recognised, and more frequently deemed as needing diagnosis, requiring precise localisation, than small volumes of ascites. Despite the paucity of experimental investigations, it makes intuitive sense to use ultrasound, if it is available, to make sure that a fluid collection is present, and that there is unimpeded access to it. One small study has shown that in a significant minority of cases, this may not be so.

Procedure

Considerations regarding the use of the "one-step" or "two-step" technique will depend on the clinical setting and the sonographic findings on a preliminary scan. The former, using real-time sonographic guidance, is more likely to be chosen with smaller volumes of ascitic fluid, or with close proximity of bowel. The two-step approach,

more easily performed without assistance, may be preferable if these constraints do not apply. With the two-step procedure, the optimal site for tap is sonographically identified and the skin marked, as described for localisation of abscesses. Usual care is taken to avoid the inferior epigastric arteries, which may be located with colour-flow Doppler, if available. The location and size of the bladder should be noted. The distance from the skin to the parietal peritoneum should be measured, for choice of needle and depth of insertion. The skin is prepped and draped, and paracentesis performed as described in detail elsewhere.[28]

Complications, as noted, are rare, and include intraperitoneal haemorrhage, abdominal wall haematomata, fluid leak, abdominal wall infections, and peritonitis.

Bladder applications

The bladder is best visualised using a general abdominal ultrasound probe in the 2·5–5 MHz range, using the highest frequency which provides sufficient penetration. The probe is oriented transversely immediately cephalad to the pubic symphysis, and "rocked" in the sagittal plane, allowing the ultrasound beam to be swept systematically from the prostate to the dome of the bladder. The normal filled bladder is a roughly rectangular anechoic structure with smooth walls in the transverse plane. Other fluid-filled structures that must be differentiated from the bladder include fluid-filled loops of bowel, large ovarian cysts, abdominal wall haematomas, and ascites.

Estimating bladder volume

Evaluation of bladder dysfunction or outlet obstruction is aided by quantification of post-void residual urine. The gold standard for evaluation of bladder volume is bladder catheterisation, carrying the risks of iatrogenic infection and urethral trauma, which are especially problematic in a patient with pre-existing urinary tract dysfunction or prostatic hypertrophy. Ultrasound provides a non-invasive and quick estimate of bladder volumes while reducing patient discomfort and anxiety.

Estimation of bladder volume is inaccurate (± 30–40% of true volume) when it is nearly empty; however, in the emergency setting, precise measurements of volume are usually moot, since

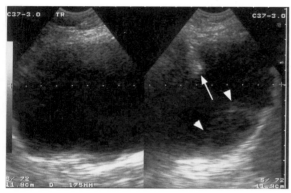

A

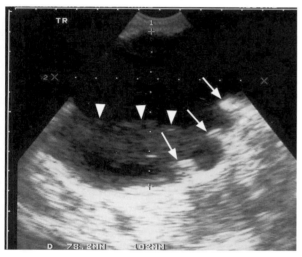

B

Figures 13.18   Sagittal and transverse views of a patient with chronic urinary retention, showing multiple trabeculae (arrows), and sediment. **(A)** shows the technique, available on most machines, of creating a composite image rather than using a "stand-off", or spacer (see Figure 13.2). The dimensions of the bladder were approximately 17·5 cm by 10 cm by 8 cm, for a volume of 1400 ml.

the qualitative information about residual volumes as "none", "small", or "large" are usually clinically sufficient. Comparisons of complex formulae to calculate bladder volume, including contour-tracing methods, have shown no advantage over simpler formulae. Simforoosh *et al*[29] evaluated 11 formulae and found one of the simplest – sagittal height multiplied by sagittal depth multiplied by transverse width – produced the most accurate results (Figure 13.18A and 13.18B).

Suprapubic aspiration and cystostomy placement

Without meticulous meatal cleansing, retraction of the foreskin or labia, and a midstream specimen,

micturition is likely to lead to contaminated urine specimens. These ideal conditions are particularly difficult to achieve in infants, especially females. In these patients, suprapubic bladder aspiration may be indicated when absolutely uncontaminated urine is necessary for diagnosis, or for the evaluation of urinary tract infection when anatomic or surgical abnormalities preclude the placement of a catheter. In adults, aspiration is indicated in males with condom catheters or phimosis (in whom the urethra and glans respectively cannot be adequately cleansed). Cystostomy tube placement is indicated for traumatic disruption of the urethra and for cases of severe urinary retention in which efforts at urethral drainage are either unsuccessful or are deemed unsafe.

Complications

Both bladder aspiration and cystostomy carry a small risk of infection, bladder injury, bowel perforation, and misplacement of the tube. These complications should be minimal with sono-graphic guidance. Ultrasound is able to demonstrate a bladder with sufficient volume to be tapped, and reduces the number of unsuccessful attempts. O'Callaghan *et al*[30] reported a success rate of 100% for first attempt suprapubic aspiration in infants following ultrasound confirmation of urine in the bladder, compared to 36% without ultrasound. Gochman *et al*[31] reported a success rate of 79% when ultrasound was used to visualise the bladder, compared to 52% without ultrasound. Both studies emphasised that first attempts at aspiration were highly successful when the bladder was full, underscoring the need for pre-hydration when aspiration is to be attempted without an ultrasound examination. As noted under "Technique" above, either the "one-step" or "two-step" techniques for sonographically identifying and accessing the bladder may be used, depending on the size of the bladder.

Ultrasound guidance in emergency cardiac procedures

Pericardiocentesis

The indication for emergency pericardiocentesis is pericardial effusion with haemodynamic compromise: that is, cardiac tamponade. The majority of large pericardial effusions do not require even elective pericardiocentesis in the absence of tamponade.

Procedure

Contrary to the usual subxiphoid approach of "blind" pericardiocentesis, ultrasound guided pericardiocentesis uses a direct transthoracic approach with much lower complication rates and higher success rates.[32,33] The patient is placed, if possible, with the head of the bed slightly elevated, and in a semi-decubitus position on the left side, to maximise cardiac contact with the chest wall. Ultrasound images are obtained, identifying the site where the effusion is thickest and most directly accessible below the probe. Ideally, a site more than 5 cm from the left sternal border should be chosen, to avoid the internal mammary artery. In addition to identifying a location for the tap, the sonographer analyses and memorises the angle and direction that needs to be taken by the pericardiocentesis needle.

Without moving the patient, the site is marked, prepped, and sterilely draped. A 10 cc syringe is partly filled with 5 cc sterile saline and attached to the hub of a 14- or 16-gauge plastic intravenous catheter (5 to 8 cm in length, depending on the thickness of the chest wall). With gentle negative pressure applied to the syringe, the needle and catheter are directed along the predetermined trajectory into the pericardial sac. Real-time sonographic information can be obtained from an adjacent window, but this is rarely necessary or practical in the management of patients with acute tamponade. Once the steel core of the intravenous needle enters the pericardial space, blood will be aspirated. Unless the ultrasound revealed a very thin layer of pericardial fluid (unlikely in the setting of tamponade), the needle is advanced 2–3 mm further, to ensure that the plastic sheath is completely through the pericardial wall and into the pericardial space. The needle is then held in place as the sheath is advanced over it. The steel core is then completely removed, thus avoiding risk of injury to the myocardium. The usual care is taken *never* to attempt to re-advance the steel needle through the plastic catheter, once it has been withdrawn, for fear of shearing off the catheter. The plastic catheter is connected to a drainage bag, and the pericardial fluid aspirated using a syringe attached to a three-way stopcock.

If pericardial drainage is not successful, or stops, the location of the catheter can be checked by direct visualisation or by use of a bedside sonographic contrast agent. This can be created by squirting 5–10 cc of saline back and forth between two partly filled syringes by way of a three-way stopcock. This aerated solution is then introduced through the catheter. If it is in the correct location, the contrast agent will be seen entering the pericardium. Subsequent management of the catheter, and techniques for its replacement by other drainage catheters using the Seldinger technique, are beyond the scope of this chapter, but described elsewhere.[32] Complications of this technique in large series are very rare. They include haemothorax, pneumothorax, bacterial pericarditis, and failure of drainage. A technique using a probe-mounted needle has also been shown to be equally successful, but since such equipment is unavailable in most emergency care settings, it is not described here.

Pacemaker placement

Elective transvenous pacemaker placement is usually accomplished with the assistance of fluoroscopy. This modality is typically neither available nor practicable for critically ill patients in need of emergent pacing. In these patients, successful pacemaker capture is often unsuccessful, leading to the uncertainty as to whether the absence of capture is due to the probe being in the wrong place, or due to a refractory heart. Studies of pacemaker placement using ultrasound guidance are limited, but several case series have attested to the utility of ultrasound to identify the pacemaker wire, its location, and electromechanical capture, when it occurs.[34–37] Any of the commonly used cardiac windows can be used.

Summary

The ability of ultrasound to provide information about soft tissues makes it a useful tool both in the diagnosis of pathological conditions and for subsequent invasive therapy, if indicated. With real-time spatial information, the guesswork is taken out of many traditionally "blind" procedures, rendering them safer, faster, and more efficacious.

Pearls and pitfalls in the evaluation of soft tissue inflammation

- Systematic methodical scanning in at least two orthogonal planes
- Compare symptomatic area with contralateral "normal" area
- Consider possibility of occult foreign body

Cellulitis versus abscess

- Optimise and vary frequency, dynamic range, gain, and focus

Apparently negative ultrasound evaluation for abscess

- Consider the possibility of iso- or hyperechoic abscess
  Look for posterior enhancement
  Look for fluid "flow" with digital or probe pressure
  Use colour flow Doppler if available
- Consider fasciitis, pyomyositis, or osteomyelitis

Evaluation of swelling around joints

- Determine whether intra- or extra-articular process
- Compare with contralateral side
- Manipulate joint to optimise view of effusion

References

1 Lammers RL. Soft Tissue Foreign Bodies. *Ann Emerg Med* 1988;**17**:1336–47.

2 Anderson MA, Newmeyer WL, Kilgore ES. Diagnosis and Treatment of Retained Foreign Bodies in the Hand. *Am J Surg* 1982;**144**:63–7.

3 Schlager D. The Use of Ultrasound in the Emergency Department. *Emerg Med Clin North Am* 1997;**15**:896–912.

4 Hill R, Conron R, Greissinger P, Heller M. Ultrasound for the Detection of Foreign Bodies in Human Tissue. *Ann Emerg Med* 1997;**29**:353–6.

5 Rockett MS, Gentile SC, Gudas CJ, Brage ME, Zygmunt KH. The use of ultrasonography for the detection of retained wooden foreign bodies in the foot. *J Foot Ankle Surg* 1995;**34(5)**:478–84.

6 Manthey DE, Storrow AB, Milbourn JM, Wagner BJ. Ultrasound Versus Radiography in the Detection of Soft-Tissue Foreign Bodies. *Ann Emerg Med* 1996;**28**:7–9.

7 Orlinsky M, Knitel P, Feit T, Chan L, Mandavia D. The comparative accuracy of radiolucent foreign body detection using ultrasonography. *Am J Emerg Med* 2000;**18**:401–3.

8 Shiels WE, Babcock DS, Wilson JL, Burch RA. Localization and guided removal of soft-tissue foreign bodies with sonography. *Am J Roentgenol* 1990;**155**:1277–81.

9 Schlager D, Sanders AB, Wiggins D, Boren W. Ultrasound for the Detection of Foreign Bodies. *Ann Emerg Med* 1991;**20(2)**:189–191.

10 Bray PW, Mahoney JL, Campbell JP. Sensitivity and specificity of ultrasound diagnosis of foreign bodies of the hand. *J Hand Surg* 1995;**20A**:661–6.

11 Gilbert FJ, Campbell RSD, Bayliss AP. The Role of Ultrasound in the Detection of Non-Radiopaque FBs. *Clin Radiol* 1990;**41**:109–12.

12 Craig JG. Infection: ultrasound-guided procedures. *Radiologic Clin North Am* 1999;**37(4)**:669–78.

13 Dean AJ, Gronczewski CA, Costantino TG. Technique for emergency medicine bedside ultrasound identification of a radiolucent foreign body. *J Emerg Med* 2003;**24(3)**:303–8.

14 Haeggstrom A, Gustafsson O, Engquist S, Engstrom CF. Intraoral ultrasonography in the diagnosis of peritonsillar abscess. *Otolaryngology* 1993;**108(3)**:243–7.

15 Scott PM, Loftus WK, Kew J, Ahuja A, Yue V, van Hasselt CA. Diagnosis of peritonsillar infections: a prospective study of ultrasound, computerized tomography and clinical diagnosis. *J Laryngol Otol* 1999;**113(3)**:229–32.

16 Kew J, Ahuja A, Loftus WK, Scott PM, Metreweli C. Peritonsillar abscess appearance on intra-oral ultrasonography. *Clin Radiol* 1998;**53(2)**:143–6.

17 Lew DP, Waldvogel FA. Osteomyelitis. *N Engl J Med* 1997;**336(14)**:999–1007.

18 Valley VT, Stahmer SA. Targeted musculoarticular sonography in the detection of joint effusions. *Acad Emerg Med* 2001;**8(4)**:361–7.

19 Chan YL, Cheng JC, Metreweli C. Sonographic evaluation of hip effusion in children. Improved visualization with the hip in extension and abduction. *Acta Radiologica* 1997;**38(5)**:867–9.

20 Berman L, Fink AM, Wilson D, McNally E. Technical note: identifying and aspirating hip effusions. *Br J Radiol* 1995;**68(807)**:306–10.

21 Bickerstaff DR, Neal LM, Booth AJ, Brennan PO, Bell MJ. Ultrasound examination of the irritable hip. *J Bone Joint Surg [Br]* 1990;**72(4)**:549–53.

22 Lichtenstein D, Hulot JS, Rabiller A, Tostivint I, Meziere G. Feasibility and safety of ultrasound-aided thoracentesis in mechanically ventilated patients. *Intens Care Med* 1999;**25(9)**:955–8.

23 Petersen S, Freitag M, Albert W, Tempel S, Ludwig K. Ultrasound-guided thoracentesis in surgical intensive care patients. *Intens Care Med* 1999;**25(9)**:1029.

24 Harnsberger HR, Lee TG, Mukuno DH. Rapid, inexpensive real-time directed thoracentesis. *Radiology* 1983;**146(2)**:545–6.

25 Matsumata T, Kanematsu T, Sugimachi K. Ultrasonically guided pleural tap. *Int Surg* 1991;**76(3)**:172–3.

26 Capizzi SA, Prakash UB. Chest roentgenography after outpatient thoracentesis. *Mayo Clin Proc* 1998;**73(10)**:948–50.

27 Bard C, Lafortune M, Breton G. Ascites: ultrasound guidance or blind paracentesis? *Can Med Assoc J* 1986;**135(3)**:209–10.

28 Marx JA. Peritoneal procedures. In: Roberts JR, Hedges JR, eds. *Clinical Procedures in Emergency Medicine.* Philadelphia: Saunders 1998, 733–49.

29 Simforoosh N, Dadkhah F, Hosseini SY, *et al.* Accuracy of residual urine measurement in men: comparison between real-time ultrasonography and catheterization. *J Urol* 1997;**158**:59–61.

30 O'Callaghan C, McDougall PN. Successful suprapubic aspiration of urine. *Arch Dis Child* 1987;**62**:1072–3.

31 Gochman RF, Karasic RB, Heller MB. Use of ultrasound to assist urine collection by suprapubic aspiration. *Ann Emerg Med* 1991;**20**:631–5.

32 Tsang TS, Freeman WK, Sinak LJ, Seward JB. Echocardiographically guided pericardiocentesis: evolution and state-of-the-art technique. *Mayo Clin Proc* 1998;**73(7)**:647–52.

33 Salem K, Mulji A, Lonn E. Echocardiographically guided pericardiocentesis – the gold standard for the management of pericardial effusion and cardiac tamponade. *Can J Cardiol* 1999;**15(11)**:1251–5.

34 Lee MS, Evans SJ, Blumberg S, Bodenheimer MM, Roth SL. Echocardiographically guided electrophysiologic testing in pregnancy. *J Amer Soc Echocardiog* 1994;**7(2)**:182–6.

35 Macedo W Jr, Sturmann K, Kim JM, Kang J. Ultrasonographic guidance of transvenous pacemaker insertion in the emergency department: a report of three cases. *J Emerg Med* 1999; **17(3)**:491–6.

36 Aguilera PA, Durham BA, Riley DA. Emergency transvenous cardiac pacing placement using ultrasound guidance. *Ann Emerg Med* 2000;**36(3)**:224–7.

37 Ettin D, Cook T. Using ultrasound to determine external pacer capture. *J Emerg Med* 1999;**17(6)**:1007–9.

14 Ultrasound in austere and mass casualty settings

LEONARD J KING

Objectives
- To describe the use of ultrasound in austere clinical environments including remote civilian practice, military deployment, and humanitarian operations
- To review the role of ultrasound in trauma and mass casualty situations

Introduction

Medical ultrasound is a well established diagnostic technique in many clinical scenarios, and an ultrasound scanner can now be regarded as a routine piece of equipment in almost every imaging department. Historically the use of ultrasound has been predominantly by radiologists, sonographers, cardiologists, and vascular/cardiac technicians in the secondary care setting. Improvements in ultrasound technology, reduction in the cost of entry level machines and increasing recognition that other medical personnel with limited application-specific training can usefully employ ultrasound as a focussed diagnostic tool, has resulted in a more widespread use of ultrasound in a variety of clinical settings. It is now commonplace for non-radiologist, hospital based clinicians to employ ultrasound in their daily practice, for example in the field of obstetrics, and in anaesthetics where ultrasound is advocated for assisting in the placement of central lines. Some primary care physicians are also performing ultrasound examinations in their own surgeries. Furthermore the easy portability of some ultrasound scanners now allows examinations to be performed outside the confines of a traditional medical facility and is proving itself to be a useful tool in a number of more austere settings, some examples of which will be discussed in this chapter.

Use of ultrasound in geographically remote locations

Medical staff practising in geographically remote locations may not have the benefit of easy access to high quality secondary care facilities including a well equipped imaging department. Obvious examples include physicians who provide primary care in Alaska or the Australian outback, medical officers on mountain or polar expeditions, and astronauts on manned space flights as an extreme example. In these situations ultrasound is an attractive imaging modality, which can be employed by non-radiologists without concerns regarding the use of ionising radiation. It is not surprising therefore that the use of ultrasound by primary care physicians is becoming increasingly popular throughout the UK particularly in rural settings such as in the Scottish highlands and islands.

Suggested benefits of general practitioners performing their own scans include:

- patients not having to travel to hospital
- no wait for an appointment
- no wait for results to be sent out
- early diagnosis
- initiation of immediate treatment
- reduced patient anxiety.[1]

It is also suggested that scanning by general practitioners is cost effective and represents an effective use of resources.[1] This will only be true however if the equipment is in frequent use, high levels of diagnostic accuracy can be sustained, and the provision of an ultrasound service does not have a negative impact on other services. What is clear however is that this practice is particularly attractive for remote primary care facilities where the time and expense involved in travelling are a major issue. Cost effectiveness can also be improved by purchasing a low cost, entry level scanner suited to the limited requirements and thus keeping the initial capital outlay to a minimum.

Scanning by primary care physicians has potential advantages for the evaluation of non-urgent cases such as assessment of bladder emptying or uncomplicated right upper quadrant pain and also for more acute patients particularly related to obstetrics and possibly trauma. This can assist in determining the necessity and/or urgency of patient transfer to a better-equipped facility. However, whilst reasonable competence in performing FAST examinations can be achieved in a few days,[2-4] there is a far greater learning curve for other ultrasound applications.

The Royal College of General Practitioners and Royal College of Radiologists joint working party report of 1993 suggested a framework for GP training in ultrasound and indicated which examinations may be appropriately carried out by GPs.[6]

Ultrasound examinations appropriately carried out in general practice by appropriately trained primary care physicians

Obstetrics
First trimester pregnancy dating
Number of fetuses and viability
Presentation
Placental site
Early pregnancy problems – pain and bleeding (but not exclusion of ectopic pregnancy)

Non-obstetric
Abdominal aortic aneurysm screening
Gallbladder and some renal tract examinations
Location of lost IUCDs

The key issue with this application of ultrasound is to ensure that adequate training has been undertaken and that individuals recognise the limits of their own skills and of ultrasound as a diagnostic technique in each clinical scenario. Whilst many accurate and clinically relevant diagnoses are being made by primary care physicians, patients with false positive examinations and incorrect interpretation of ultrasound signs by inexperienced operators are not infrequently encountered. In the author's own experience, this rarely results in significant harm to the patient whose secondary care may well have been expedited by an apparently positive scan, except where confirmatory imaging by an experienced operator has not been performed. Of greater concern however is the false negative examination, which results in inappropriate reassurance, or where symptoms are incorrectly attributed to what is an incidental·finding such as gallstones.

It is important therefore that where possible, scans by inexperienced operators, which demonstrate significant findings, are confirmed by an experienced operator prior to definitive management. It is also imperative that the ultrasound findings are considered within the context of each patient's clinical status and that undue reliance is not placed on a negative ultrasound examination. If clinical doubt remains after an apparently normal scan then further advice should be sought. Teleradiology is an attractive option for providing further advice in such cases if robust links with an enthusiastic imaging department can be established.

Use of ultrasound on military operations

Ultrasound is a well established, deployable asset for use on military operations, but until recently has only been suitable for use on larger scale operations where the deployment of a radiologist or ultrasound trained technician could be justified. In such situations there is a steady demand for ultrasound from surgeons and physicians. During a recent military peacekeeping deployment, ultrasound comprised around 4% of imaging requests to the radiology department of a field hospital where plain radiography and computed tomography (CT) were also available.

Referrals for ultrasound in the field hospital setting can be highly variable and are not just related to trauma. In addition to general abdominal and pelvic scanning, including the assessment of early pregnancy problems, there are frequent requests for musculoskeletal, testicular, and vascular ultrasound plus occasional patients with suspected appendicitis in whom the clinical evaluation is equivocal. It is thus important that both low frequency (3–5Mhz) curvilinear and high frequency (10MHz or greater) linear probes are available. High frequency linear array probes can be obtained for most ultrasound machines including portable scanners, and in general a machine with interchangeable probes is the preferred option for field use rather than a less expensive machine with a single fixed transducer.

Experience from several mass casualty situations dealt with by military field hospitals in the Balkans has confirmed the benefits of trauma ultrasound in the hands of trained radiologists and sonographers (Figures 14.1 and 14.2). It is now recognised however that surgeons and other medically qualified personnel can be trained to detect free thoracic or peritoneal fluid using a

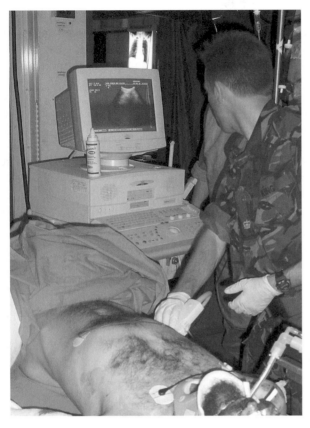

Figure 14.1 A military radiologist performing a FAST examination with a platform mounted US scanner on a mine strike victim.

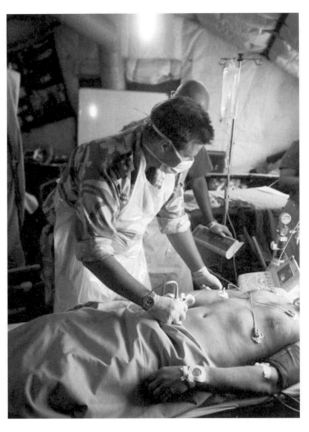

Figure 14.2 A FAST trained military surgeon utilising handheld ultrasound to assess a casualty with blunt abdominal trauma in a field hospital environment.

focussed technique (FAST)[2–4,7–13] and robust, portable, and relatively inexpensive ultrasound machines have now been developed. Thus ultrasound has become a viable tool for deployment in a wider variety of military operations such as with small field surgical teams, on board Navy ships, or on medical evacuation flights. With this in mind a course in FAST ultrasound has been developed for UK military surgeons who are now using the technique to assess casualties when no support from a sonographer or radiologist is available. Ongoing developments in teleradiology capability also allow ultrasound images obtained by non-radiologists to be viewed remotely by more experienced clinicians at a base location, who can then offer further advice.

One of the major problems with imaging equipment in field hospital use is the ability to function effectively in a hostile environment. This is a particular problem for CT, which although a valuable tool for the assessment of trauma patients, can suffer from reliability problems, for example due to dust in the slip

rings. It is also sensitive to vibration from exploding ordnance plus extremes of ambient temperature. All CT scanners will only operate when the x ray tube is within a specific temperature range and scanning will be temporarily suspended if the tube temperature rises above its maximum due to heat produced as a by-product of x ray generation. Whilst this is becoming a relatively minor problem in hospital practice with modern scanners in air conditioned hospital departments it is certainly a factor which can affect scanning in the field if heat dispersal is hampered by high ambient temperatures.

Conversely CT scanners require a tube warm-up period of around 20 minutes before clinical images can be obtained. In a hospital department during normal working hours this is not usually a significant problem as most scanners are in almost constant use, but out of hours and in field hospital conditions this can be a cause of delay. By comparison ultrasound machines tend to be more robust, with manufacturers' quoted working temperature ranges of approximately

10–40°C, although the components of at least one commercially available portable scanner have been tested to well below this range. Ultrasound probes however are rather fragile and the transducer crystals may break if knocked or dropped onto a hard surface. Platform mounted scanners can also be damaged when moving between wards and departments. For example transducer cables may become entangled in the wheels causing damage, or probes and poorly mounted monitors can be dislodged, particularly when traversing ramps or negotiating uneven surfaces, which are a feature of field hospitals.

Providing adequate servicing and maintenance of imaging equipment is another major issue for field hospital imaging departments. Military medical physics personnel can be given sufficient training to carry out basic maintenance procedures and effect repairs to relatively simple problems. Diagnostic analysis of CT problems can also be affected by a telephone link up to the system manufacturer or by connecting to a laptop computer with appropriate software. Military technicians do not always deploy with a small field hospital however, and if present they may be unable to deal with major problems involving imaging equipment, which would then require the services of an engineering representative from the manufacturer. These civilian technicians may be unable or unwilling to carry out repairs within a forward area of operations for a variety of reasons and it is significantly easier to backload a portable ultrasound machine to a rear area for repair or replacement than most other items of imaging hardware. Ultrasound machines also tend to require less frequent maintenance than other equipment, particularly CT. Thus ultrasound has clear advantages over other imaging equipment for deployment into inaccessible areas.

One further advantage of portable ultrasound over other imaging equipment is that it can be used effectively within minutes of deploying into the field and can be quickly packed away. This makes it a very effective tool for use in a rapidly changing tactical situation where deployment or relocation may be required at short notice.

Use of ultrasound on humanitarian operations

Humanitarian medical operations by non-government organisations (NGOs) provide a valuable service both as ongoing healthcare providers in underdeveloped areas with poor healthcare infrastructure and on disaster relief operations. Most of the problems and issues relating to the use of ultrasound in remote civilian practice and on military operations are equally relevant to NGOs. Care of patients can be hampered by the limited availability of imaging facilities in remote locations and ultrasound would appear to be a cost effective option for extending their imaging capability. Portable ultrasound scanners in particular are being recognised as a valuable tool in this situation and whilst little published data is available on the outcome of such ventures, there is certainly anecdotal evidence of its usefulness from a number of respected individuals and organisations.

Use of ultrasound in the trauma/mass casualty setting

Focussed ultrasound has now become a standard technique in many trauma centres for assessing trauma patients in the accident and emergency/trauma room environment, particularly in the United States and some parts of Europe. A key factor in this increasing use is the easy portability of the recently developed compact, lightweight machines, which combine good technical performance with genuine handheld capability. Gaining adequate access to a multi-trauma patient undergoing resuscitation procedures with a bulky platform based machine can be difficult, as can obtaining a suitable power supply. These problems are particularly pronounced in the sub-optimal conditions of a field hospital environment, where power supplies may be unreliable, electrical sockets are limited and in high demand for other medical equipment, and transformers may be required to convert between different voltages in multinational medical facilities. Use of a portable, battery powered ultrasound scanner significantly improves this situation without a significant reduction in diagnostic performance compared with a conventional, platform-mounted ultrasound machine.[14] Technological advances in probe design have resulted in the availability of small footprint, curvilinear probes for use with portable scanners, which provide optimal visualisation through relatively small acoustic windows. This can be of significant benefit when probe access is limited by residual clothing, dressings, ECG leads, and in situ thoracocentesis tubes. In the author's experience, several patients can be scanned using a hand held machine in the time taken for scanning one patient with a conventional platform-mounted machine, due to the above factors.

Ultrasound can be performed concurrently with other resuscitation procedures in a resuscitation area and the results are known within a few minutes of the patient's arrival in hospital, if equipment and a suitably trained individual are immediately available. This contrasts with CT where patients, and often several of the attending staff, require to be moved from the resuscitation area to the scan room and other procedures temporarily suspended. Even with modern multislice scanners and experienced staff this can be a time consuming process and is not recommended for unstable patients following thoracoabdominal trauma. In the mass casualty situation this time factor becomes even more significant as multiple patients require rapid assessment and CT may be in high demand for head and spine imaging.[15]

As no ionising radiation is involved, ultrasound can be readily repeated at frequent intervals if necessary and in the vicinity of other patients and medical personnel without concerns over radiation safety. This makes the technique ideal for use as a triaging tool, which can be taken from patient to patient in a makeshift triage area. A good example of this was the 1988 Armenian earthquake disaster where sonography was performed as the primary screening procedure in 400 of 750 casualties admitted to the hospital within a 72-hour period.[15] In the Armenian experience, ultrasound was performed on patients in temporary examination rooms, which were set up in a hospital reception area, or at the bedside immediately after admission. A combination of two platform-mounted ultrasound scanners and two desktop portable scanners on trolleys that could be moved to the bedside was used with an average examination time of four minutes. Pathology was demonstrated in 12·8% of patients, with a 1% false negative rate and no false positives. Thus ultrasound proved to be a rapid and accurate method for demonstrating abdominal injuries in this large group of patients, including those with retroperitoneal trauma.

Use of ultrasound in the mass casualty situation is not restricted to hospital use as the more portable, handheld, battery operated machines now available can also be easily deployed to an incident scene to assist in the triaging of multiple casualties for evacuation. Ultrasound images are optimally viewed in low ambient light conditions, which may not be achievable in this clinical setting, particularly during daylight in open air conditions, but virtual reality style viewing goggles can be used in conjunction with a hand held scanner which eliminates this problem.

Although primarily used for the detection of thoracic and abdominal free fluid in the acute trauma situation, ultrasound can, in experienced hands, demonstrate visceral injuries, pneumothoraces,[16] extremity injuries including fractures,[17] and some vascular injuries, including post traumatic pseudoaneurysms and arteriovenous fistulae. These types of application however require substantially more training than a basic FAST examination.

Summary

Ultrasound is a relatively inexpensive, robust, and flexible tool the use of which can be easily extended into a variety of austere clinical circumstances. There are a number of clear advantages of ultrasound, particularly portable ultrasound, over other imaging equipment particularly with regard to cost, portability, and robustness. The exact role of ultrasound and its clinical effectiveness in each clinical scenario is dependent on the training and experience of the operator. It is likely that the use of ultrasound as a focussed tool by a wide range of medical personnel will continue to expand and become commonplace outside the confines of a hospital imaging department.

References

1 Hussain P, Melville D, Mannings R, Curry D, Kay D, Ford P. Evaluation of a training and diagnostic ultrasound service for general practitioners using narrowband ISDN. *J Telemed Telecare* 1999;**5**:S1 95–9.

2 Thomas B, Falcone RE, Vasquez D, *et al.* Ultrasound evaluation of blunt abdominal trauma: programme implementation, initial experience and learning curve. *J Trauma* 1997;**42**:384–90.

3 Shackford SR, Rogers FB, Osler TM, Trabulsy ME, Clauss DV, Vane DW. Focussed abdominal sonogram for trauma: the learning curve of non-radiologist clinicians in detecting haemoperitoneum. *J Trauma* 1999;**46**:553–64.

4 Salen PN, Melanson SW, Heller MB. The Focused Sonography for Trauma (FAST) Examination: Considerations and Recommendations for Training Physicians in the Use of a New Clinical Tool. *Acad Emerg Med* 2000;**7(2)**:162–8.

5 The Royal College of Radiologists. *Guidance for the Training in Ultrasound of Medical Non-Radiologists*, 1997.

6 The Royal College of General Practitioners and The Royal College of Radiologists. *Basic Ultrasound Training for General Practitioners – Report of a joint working party*. London: The Royal College of Radiologists and The Royal College of General Practitioners, January 1993.

7 Ma OJ, Mateer JR, Ogata M, Kefer MP, Whittmann D, Aprahamian C. Prospective analysis of a rapid trauma ultrasound examination performed by emergency physicians. *J Trauma* 1995;**38**:879–85.

8 Ingeman JE, Plewa MC, Okasinsyi RE, King RW, Knotts FB. Emergency physician use of ultrasonography in blunt abdominal trauma. *Acad Emerg Med* 1996;**3**:931–7.

9 Rozycki GS, Feliciano DV, Schmidt JA, *et al.* The role of surgeon performed ultrasound in patients with possible cardiac wounds. *Ann Surg* 1996;**223**:737–46.

10 Rozycki GS, Ballard RB, Feliciano DV, Schmidt JA, Pennington SD. Surgeon performed ultrasound for the assessment of truncal injuries. *Ann Surg* 1998;**228**:557–67.

11 Rozycki G. Surgeon performed ultrasound: its use in clinical practice. *Ann Surg* 1998;**228**:16–28.

12 Smith RS, Kern SJ, Fry WR, Helmer SD. Institutional learning curve of surgeon performed trauma ultrasound. *Arch Surg* 1998;**133**:530–6.

13 Brooks A, Davies B, Connolly J. Prospective evaluation of hand held ultrasound in the diagnosis of blunt abdominal trauma. *J Army Med Corps* 2002;**148**:19–21.

14 Kirkpatrick AW, Simons RK, Brown R, Nicolaou S, Dulchavsky S. The hand-held FAST: experience with hand-held trauma sonography in a level-I urban trauma center. *Injury* 2002;**33**:303–8.

15 Sarkisian AE, Khondkarian RA, Amirbekian NM, Bagdasarian NB, Khojayan RL, Oganesian YT. Sonographic screening of mass casualties for abdominal and renal injuries following the 1988 Armenian earthquake. *J Trauma* 1991;**31**:247–50.

16 Dulchavsky SA, Schwarz KL, Kirkpatrick AW, *et al.* Prospective Evaluation of Thoracic Ultrasound in the Detection of Pneumothorax. *J Trauma* 2001;**50**: 201–5.

17 Dulchavsky SA, Henry SE, Moed BR, *et al.* Advanced ultrasonic diagnosis of extremity trauma: the FASTER examination. *J Trauma* 2002;**53**:28–32.

Further reading

Guidance on the use of ultrasound locating devices for placing central venous catheters. London: National Institute for Clinical Excellence, September 2002. Can also be read at http://www.nice.org.uk/Docref. asp?d=36753 (accessed December 2003).

http://www.sonosite.com

15 Training in emergency ultrasound

SUSIE HEWITT, MICHAEL R MAROHN, DAVID WHERRY

Objectives
To review
- The emerging role of ultrasound as an adjunct to emergency care
- Established models of training
- The potential for developing competency based training in the UK

Introduction

The value of ultrasound as an extension of clinical diagnosis is becoming recognised by many doctors providing emergency care throughout the world. The availability of portable hand-held devices has enhanced the availability of ultrasound at the point of care of critically ill patients. Ultrasound continues to cross the boundaries between specialties and emergency medicine joins the increasing number of non-radiology specialties which employ ultrasound as an adjunct to clinical examination.

Ultrasound is a very rapidly evolving technology and its performance is demanding and operator dependent with risks of misinterpretation. It therefore opens the possibility of medical legal liability. Demonstrating competence in a clinical skill is an essential part of clinical governance, particularly when the skill has been traditionally associated with a specific specialty. In the climate of governance and potential sensitivities between disciplines, the role of training assumes particular importance. Ultrasound courses for non-radiology specialists are available in the United Kingdom and are accredited by various bodies for continued professional development. However there is no national lead in developing and maintaining competence specifically to meet the needs of those providing emergency care.

This contrasts with progress in America and Australia where ultrasound is established as an adjunct to emergency care. Rozycki *et al* have demonstrated the effectiveness of ultrasound in the management of the trauma patient.[1-4] The American College of Emergency Physicians (ACEP) and the Australasian College for Emergency Medicine (ACEM) specifically support the use of ultrasound imaging by emergency physicians for at least the following primary indications:

- traumatic haemoperitoneum
- abdominal aortic aneurysm
- pericardial fluid
- ectopic pregnancy
- evaluation of renal and biliary tract disease.

Both the ACEP and ACEM have published policy statements on credentialing.[5,6]

This Chapter will focus on the American experience to date in developing training programmes and credentialing systems, and describe how these might form a basis for progress in the UK and elsewhere. Many of the training issues that have been addressed by general surgeons in America are applicable in considering how to move forward in training for non-radiology specialists involved in emergency care.

An American perspective

The American Board of Surgery has required surgeons to have exposure to surgical ultrasound since 1995. There are a large number of physicians who need postgraduate training in the use of ultrasound and the American College of Surgeons (ACS) has taken the lead role in educating and encouraging surgeons to perform ultrasound to improve patient care. Three aspects of training have emerged: verification, certification, and credentialing.

Verification

The American College of Surgeons Committee on Emerging Surgical Technology and Education (CESTE) established the National Ultrasound Faculty (NUF) with the mission to develop a surgical education programme. The goal of the ultrasound education programme is to train surgeons in the effective use of ultrasound for specific surgical problems and/or diseases. The ACS provides verification in ultrasound training. It documents attendance at courses provided by the ACS and documents successful testing in both a written and practical examination. It does not document ultrasound experience, outcomes, or maintenance of skills. Initially, the College set up a National Ultrasound Faculty and an Ultrasound Imaging Group (UIG). Recently, these two groups were combined into a single NUF.

The ACS ultrasound training programme is modelled on the Advanced Trauma Life Support (ATLS) course.[7] The training is based on the concept of basic and advanced modules. The basic module is a prerequisite for all the advanced courses and emphasises ultrasound physics, instrumentation, scanning techniques, and interpretation including pitfalls. Advanced courses are divided into the following modules:

- acute care setting
- abdominal ultrasound (trans-abdominal, intra-operative, laparoscopic)
- breast ultrasound
- head and neck ultrasound
- vascular ultrasound
- rectal ultrasound.

The Basic and Advanced courses are held each year at the annual and spring meetings of the ACS. In addition, the College has exported these courses to several surgical societies and institutions. Exporting a course requires the identification of a course director who must be a member of the NUF, together with instructors, certified by the ACS. The type of ultrasound course must be specified and approval of the course should be obtained from the Vice-Chairman for Education of the ACS.

The ACS provides materials and manuals in a similar way to ATLS. The course must comply with a ratio of five students to one instructor. Courses and manuals are standardised (as with ATLS) and carefully developed and updated by the NUF. At the end of the course the student must pass a written and practical examination with a grade of at least 80%. The ACS documents attendance at the course and successful testing and the student is awarded a certificate of verification.

The basic module runs over a period of four hours. The content is solely academic without a hands-on portion and concludes with a written test. The advanced modules vary in length of time depending on which module the student is

attending. All advanced modules include an academic as well as a hands-on portion and conclude with both a written and practical test.

Certification

Surgical specialist societies have worked with the NUF and the ACS in developing educational courses and materials. The ACS encourages specialist societies to develop ultrasound performance guidelines for verification and certification. Certification, as opposed to verification of training, is a more demanding and involved process. The guidelines for certification in breast ultrasound are well developed and are described here as an example of the certification process.

The American Society of Breast Surgeons (ASBS) has recently developed its requirements for breast ultrasound certification. It provides a framework for the general principles pertaining to the proper performance and interpretation of diagnostic ultrasound and the appropriate application of ultrasound-guided interventions. A summary of the entire application process is as follows:

1 submission of candidate information and payment of fees
2 eligibility criteria
3 Continuing medical education (CME) requirements
4 equipment and quality assurance measures
5 attestations
7 code of professional practice
8 submission of clinical case reports.

The completed certification process involves both a clinical and a formal written examination, both of which must be completed successfully for certification to be awarded. They may be completed in any order within a 12-month period. The application for certification includes submission of clinical cases and hard copy images. It is designed to elicit information that clearly and accurately represents the surgeon's training, clinical experience, and quality assurance practices. The information and documentation submitted by each applicant is evaluated on the basis of designated criteria. One condition of eligibility for certification is that each candidate agrees to comply with the ASBS' standards, policies, and procedures. Membership of the ASBS is not required for certification.

In addition the candidate must sign an attestation form that a minimum procedure volume has been achieved. The requirements are as follows.

- A minimum annual procedure volume of 100 mammography examinations, including a review of authenticated reports.
- A minimum of 80 diagnostic and 20 interventional ultrasound cases.
- The applicant must demonstrate that he or she has a firm grasp of image interpretation, can accurately describe findings, perform appropriate interventions based on the clinical and imaging data, and appropriately use the results of the intervention to guide further management.
- Documentation of 10 specific cases must be done from the required minimum of 100 breast ultrasound examinations performed within the last 12 months. The 10 cases must be submitted for review with the application and must include five diagnostic cases and five interventional cases. Among the interventional cases, three must be core biopsies and two must be cyst aspirations or fine needle aspiration biopsies. Ultrasound guided, vacuum assisted, or rotational core biopsy procedures may be submitted in place of core biopsy procedures.

Each of the 10 cases submitted must include a hard copy of the ultrasound images and a copy of the procedure note and any relevant pathology reports. The indication for the procedure should be noted together with the clinical outcome or plan for further assessment.

Once awarded, certification is only valid for five years before the process must be repeated.

As can be seen from this example, certification is a demanding process that should be led by a specialist body.

Credentialing

The American system for credentialing is department specific and performed at local hospital level. Credentialing is frequently stratified according to the level of difficulty in obtaining and interpreting images.

Level 1 credentialing is required for the acute care module and can be awarded by the hospital after the physician has attended an appropriate training course. The process requires written verification, by the ACS, of attendance and

successful completion of the basic and advanced acute care module. The applicant is then proctor or mentor ready. The mentor can be a radiologist, a physician, or a surgeon competent in acute care ultrasound. Prospective studies have shown that after approximately 25 mentored examinations most students are capable of performing acute care ultrasound independently, and prospective studies have shown that surgeons who perform FAST examinations have a sensitivity of 93% and a specificity of 98.7% comparing favourably with radiologists with 90% for sensitivity and 99·2% for specificity.[1–4,8,9]

In order for the hospital to act favourably on credentialing, evidence of verified training by the ACS is needed and the mentor is required to sign off the candidate as competent.

Level 2 credentialing would be applied to more complex ultrasound procedures such as breast and hepato-biliary ultrasound. An example of certification in breast ultrasound has been outlined above and it is a good standard by which credentialing could be granted. Credentialing requires formal training and experience, uniform standards, determination of competence, and monitored performance. The granting of privileges is for a limited time and requires a mechanism for their renewal.

Practical advice on getting started

Getting started
- Complete a basic and advanced course
- Identify a mentor or proctor preferably in your own department
- Document all procedures and then compare outcomes with the mentor

Getting started requires access to ultrasound machines, patients, and most of all, experience and guidance. Ultrasound machines are frequently already available in the hospital environment, such as in radiology, cardiology emergency room, vascular surgery, and urology. Ultrasound machines can be purchased if need be by sharing costs with other specialists such as vascular, colo-rectal, urology, and neurosurgery. Much can be learned from every ultrasound scan; for example, in doing an acute care or FAST examination, familiarity with the anatomy of the liver, the kidneys, the gallbladder, the spleen, and the biliary tract are soon learned. Over time, this exposure will help to develop competence in ultrasound.

Familiarity with the language or terminology of ultrasound is required such as descriptions of echogenicity – anechoic, hypoechoic, hyperechoic, etc. Confidence in detecting ultrasound artefacts including posterior enhancement or shadowing, mirror images, the ring down effect, and the comet tail effect will be achieved over time.

A documentation form should be available for use at the time of the examination. This should capture the demographics of the patient, the findings on ultrasound with site-specific essentials, and the type of machine and transducer employed. In addition, there should be a section for the outcome to include any follow up CT scans or intra-operative findings. Finally, take every opportunity to review and compare findings with a radiologist.

Find an ultrasound machine and begin scanning
- Start simple and then add complexity
- Gradually gain experience

Ultrasound in the UK – forces for change

In the UK several groups of doctors outside the specialty of radiology are recognising the value of ultrasound as part of their clinical practice. This has prompted the Royal College of Radiologists to publish recommendations for training of non-radiology medical specialists in the use of ultrasound.[10] The College acknowledges that ultrasound scanning cannot be restricted to radiologists and cites the requirement of some European boards, such as gastro-enterology, that competence in ultrasound examination is part of the core curriculum.[11]

Recommendations on the accreditation process are made based on the syllabus of the first Fellowship of the Royal College of Radiologists' examination where it relates to ultrasound. Three hundred ultrasound examinations are expected for the completion of the first practical module, and 150 for subsequent modules. These recommendations have not been developed to support the application of ultrasound as a focussed technique to answer specific questions in

emergency care. The discrepancy between the UK and the US and Australian recommendations for training suggest a different level of competence is required for specific "rule in" examinations compared to the level of training required to confidently and accurately "rule out" pathology.

A further challenge to develop a focussed training programme has been set by the National Institute for Clinical Excellence (NICE) following the publication of technology appraisal guidance on the use of ultrasound locating devices for placing central venous catheters (CVCs).[12] This guidance is another force for change that supports the role of ultrasound as a tool that crosses boundaries between specialties. It is recognised that CVCs are inserted for a variety of indications in different settings including at the bedside in an emergency. Whilst acknowledging that experienced operators using traditional landmark methods can achieve relatively high success rates, there are risks of complications with potentially serious consequences, depending on patient factors and the circumstances of insertion.

The evidence to support the guidance is most robust for the elective placement of CVCs in the internal jugular vein in adults using 2-D ultrasound imaging. However confidence is expressed in extrapolating this analysis to ward based settings, to other sites of CVC insertion, and to CVC placement in children.

The financial and service implications of the guidance are considered in terms of equipment purchase and training sufficient numbers of competent practitioners. Maintaining competence in the landmark method is considered to be important and the guidance suggests that this technique is taught alongside the ultrasound-guided technique. The guidance supports the need to spread the necessary skills across several related disciplines to ensure that there are sufficient numbers of competent operators to support the service, particularly on an emergency basis. The Royal College of Anaesthetists has responded to the guidance and described it as fair and sensible.[13]

Training in emergency ultrasound in the UK – the next steps

The first step in securing the viability of emergency ultrasound is careful clarification of its use as a focussed technique. This will ensure that expectations are reasonable and achievable and may go some way to reassure colleagues in radiology about the limits of its application. The next step is to move forward with a competency-based framework for training that addresses the issues of verification or accreditation of training courses, certification, and credentialing. The development and accreditation of a training programme by the parent body of one or more of the stakeholders (such as the Faculty of Accident and Emergency Medicine, the Royal College of Surgeons, Royal College of Anaesthetists, or the Royal College of Radiologists) is vital to develop a programme that is educationally sound and reproducible, and will meet the needs of practitioners involved in emergency care.

Taking a national view on verification will involve the design of basic and advanced modules, developing course manuals and material, and a coordinated approach to monitoring attendance and successful completion of modules. The structure of the training programme is likely to include a mandatory generic introductory module and elective focused modules such as FAST scanning, examination for suspected abdominal aortic aneurysm, vascular access, etc. A proposal for an outline of an introductory module in emergency ultrasound and a proposed focussed module template are shown below.

Proposed contents of an introductory module in emergency ultrasound

- The biophysics of ultrasound
- Safety
- Equipment orientation
- Image quality and artefact
- Image capture and storage
- Limitations of focussed examinations
- Documentation

Proposed template for a focussed module

Course overview

- Problem based scenario with underpinning anatomy and pathology
- Psychomotor skills training with live or simulated models
- Recognition of focussed findings and pitfalls

Supervised practice

- Identification of a mentor
- Maintenance of a log book and portfolio of instructional cases

Skill maintenance and quality assurance

- Audit of personal and departmental practice
- Monitoring patient outcomes

To determine the certification process appropriate to UK practice a consideration of the eligibility criteria and minimum necessary experience is required. For specialties involved in emergency care the minimum entry requirement might be year four of a specialist registrar training programme. Methods of assessment must be considered and while a written or practical test may form part of the certification process, a logbook and portfolio of instructional cases demonstrate commitment to continued professional development and will be valuable in assessing competence. The issue of equating a defined number of scans with competence has not been investigated in the UK. However it would be reasonable to look to the American and Australian models as a start and refine this when evidence concerning skill acquisition and maintenance in the UK setting becomes available.

The use of ultrasound as a clinical decision and procedural support tool is attractive to specialties involved in emergency care and is being promoted in the UK as a specific goal-directed, focussed examination.[14] Once established the anticipated benefits to patient care such as time to diagnosis and definitive care can be formally evaluated in the UK setting. Ultrasound continues to be a rapidly evolving technology. However its performance is operator dependent and therefore not without risk. The challenge is to link the enthusiasm of non-radiology specialists with the intended benefits by a robust training programme.

Summary

An increasing number of non-radiological specialists are recognising the value of ultrasound as a clinical decision and procedural support tool. The use of ultrasound by emergency physicians as a focussed technique is established in America and Australasia underpinned by a nationally led educational programme. A system for developing and maintaining competence in ultrasound as a focussed technique is required to meet the needs of those providing emergency care in the UK.

References

1 Rozycki GS, Ochsner MG, Jaffin JH, *et al.* Prospective evaluation of surgeons' use of ultrasound in the evaluation of trauma patients. *J Trauma* 1993;**34**:516–27.

2 Rozycki GS, Ochsner MG, Schmidt JA, *et al.* A prospective study of surgeon-performed ultrasound as the primary adjuvant modality for injured patient assessment. *J Trauma* 1995;**39**:492–8.

3 Rozycki GS, Shackford SR. Ultrasound, what every trauma surgeon should know. *J Trauma* 1996;**10**: 1–4.

4 Rozycki GS, Ballard RB, Feliciano DV, *et al.* Surgeon-performed ultrasound for the assessment of truncal injuries. *Ann Surg* 1998;**228**:557–67.

5 American College of Emergency Physicians. ACEP emergency ultrasound guidelines – 2001. *Ann Emerg Med* 2001;**38**:470–81.

6 Australian College of Emergency Medicine. *Policy document – Credantialling for ED ultrasonography.* Victoria: Australian College of Emergency Medicine, 2000.

7 The American College of Surgeons. *Advanced Trauma Life Support Student Manual.* Chicago: The American College of Surgeons, 1997.

8 Shackford SR, Ricci MA, Hebert JC. Education and credentialing. *Probl Gen Surg* 1997;**14**:226–32.

9 Shackford SR, Rogers FB, Osler TM, *et al.* Focused abdominal sonogram for trauma: The learning curve of non-radiologist clinicians in detecting hemoperitoneum. *J Trauma* 1999;**46**:553–64.

10 Board of the Faculty of Clinical Radiology, Royal College of Radiologists. *Guidance for the training in ultrasound of medical non-radiologists.* London: Royal College of Radiologists, 1997.

11 European Board of Gastro-enterologists. Chapter 6. *Requirements for training in the specialty of gastro-enterology.* European training charter for medical specialists. Brussels: European union of medical specialists, 1995.

12 National Institute for Clinical Excellence Technology Appraisal No.49. *Guidance on the use of ultrasound locating devices for placing central venous catheters.* London: NICE 2000.

13 The Royal College of Anaesthetists Bulletin 17. NICE Technology Appraisal guidance No. 49. *The use of ultrasound locating devices for placing central venous catheters.* Comments from the Royal College of Anaesthetists. London: Royal College of Anaesthetists, 2003.

14 Brenchley J, Sloan JP, Thompson PK. Echoes of things to come. Ultrasound in UK emergency practice. *J Accid Emerg Med* 2000;**17**:170–5.

Further reading

1. *Ultrasound for Surgeons.* American College of Surgeons. 633 N. Clair St., Chicago, IL. 60611–3211.

2. *Breast Ultrasound Certification* (Revised 10/31/02). The American Society of Breast Surgeons. 585 Main Street, Suite 243 Laurel, Md. 20707. The application and requirements can be obtained from the AIUM at the following address: 14750 Sweitzer Lane, Suite 100, Laurel, MD 207075–906.

Index

Page numbers in **bold** type refer to figures; those in *italic* refer to tables or boxed material.